SUCCESSFUL NURSE COMMUNICATION

COMMUNICATION

Safe Care, Healthy Workplaces, & Rewarding Careers

Beth Boynton, RN, MS

Nurse Consultant

Portsmouth, New Hampshire

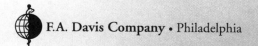

F.A. Davis Company • Philadelphia

F. A. Davis Company
1915 Arch Street
Philadelphia, PA 19103
www.fadavis.com

Printed in the United States of America

Last digit indicates print number: 10 9 8 7 6 5 4 3 2 1

Publisher, Nursing: Terri Wood Allen
Director of Content Development: Darlene D. Pedersen
Content Project Manager: Echo Gerhart; Julia Curcio
Design and Illustration Manager: Carolyn O'Brien

As new scientific information becomes available through basic and clinical research, recommended treatments and drug therapies undergo changes. The author(s) and publisher have done everything possible to make this book accurate, up to date, and in accord with accepted standards at the time of publication. The author(s), editors, and publisher are not responsible for errors or omissions or for consequences from application of the book, and make no warranty, expressed or implied, in regard to the contents of the book. Any practice described in this book should be applied by the reader in accordance with professional standards of care used in regard to the unique circumstances that may apply in each situation. The reader is advised always to check product information (package inserts) for changes and new information regarding dose and contraindications before administering any drug. Caution is especially urged when using new or infrequently ordered drugs.

Library of Congress Control Number: 2015937542

Successful Nurse Communication *is dedicated to Gabriel Summerhill.*

In his memory, I hope this book provides students with compelling reasons and strategies for communicating effectively and respectfully in order to provide the highest standard of safe and compassionate care throughout their nursing careers.

Writing a textbook for nurses is an incredible honor. As an RN for more than 25 years and a consultant for almost 10, I am excited by the opportunity to convey the expertise I have gained in communication and collaboration to nursing students all over the United States and possibly beyond. It is an amazing honor. But that is not what has motivated me to write this book.

A combination of education, nursing practice, and personal experience has led me to discover extremely important and easily overlooked connections between our ability to communicate effectively and favorable outcomes involving patient safety, the cultures in which we work, and our own health. I want all healthcare professionals and consumers to see these connections so that we can work together for positive change.

This book is dedicated to the memory of Gabriel Summerhill, a boy who died at the age of 20 months as a result of multiple medical errors. He is one of many victims of preventable death and injury in a healthcare setting. I didn't know Gabriel, but I have come to know his mother, Leilani Schweitzer, as we have crossed paths in our respective work for making healthcare safer. She, too, has seen the connections between communication and patient safety, but at a devastating price.

As human beings, we will never be perfect, but as nurses, we must be committed to providing the safest and most compassionate care possible. While doing so, we deserve to practice in workplaces that understand, respect, and support the complexity of our work. Effective and respectful communication is essential to these ideals, and this is what has motivated me to write *Successful Nurse Communication*.

Beth Boynton, RN, MS
Portsmouth, New Hampshire

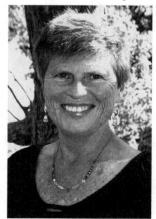

CONTRIBUTORS TO "CONFIDENT VOICES" FEATURES

Chapter 1

Renee Pontbriand, RN, ADN
Assistant Director of Nursing, Nursing
  Supervisor, Visiting Nurse, Member of
  Worldwide Leaders in Healthcare
Clipper Harbor of Portsmouth (a Genesis
  Facility)
Interim Healthcare
Portsmouth, New Hampshire
Modeling Good Behavior

**Candace (Candy) Campbell,
  DNP, RN, CNL**
Assistant Professor of Nursing and Health
  Science
University of San Francisco
San Francisco, California
As Guests in Our Patients' Home

Chapter 2

Erika Hunter, MEd
Knowledge Manager
Hewlett Packard
Lee, New Hampshire
The Benefits of Naming Emotions

Jorinda Margolis, LICSW
Private Practice
Exeter, New Hampshire
*How Compassion and Mindfulness Can
  Decrease Suffering*

Chapter 3

Briana Pefley, BSN, RN
Charge Nurse
University of Detroit Mercy
Detroit, Michigan
*The Spirit of Inquiry, Evidence-Based
  Practice, and Developing Your Innate
  Curiosity*

Pamela Neff Montembeau, PT, DPT
Physical Therapist
Kittery, Maine
Listening

Chapter 4

Patricia Iyer, MSN, RN, LRCC
President
The Pat Iyer Group
Stockton, New Jersey
Don't Let Them Down

Terri Goodman, PhD, RN, CNOR
Principal
Terri Goodman & Associates
Dallas, Texas
Welcome to the Internship

Chapter 5

Patricia Ann Bemis, RN, CEN, LHCRM
Online Course Facilitator
University of Florida
University of Central Florida
Rockledge, Florida
*A Few Mnemonics for Keeping
  Communication Orderly and Pertinent*

Robert J. Latino, B.S. BAM
CEO
Reliability Center, Inc.
Hopewell, Virginia
*Failure to Effectively Communicate: A Root
  Cause Analysis*

Chapter 6

Martine Ehrenclou, MA
Author, Healthcare Advocate
Los Angeles, California
*My Empathic Nurse and an Almost
  Unbearable Night*

Lynn McVey, MS
Chief Operating Officer
Meadowlands Hospital Medical Center
Secaucus, New Jersey
*A CEO's View of Care Coordination From
    the Inside*

Chapter 7

Alan H. Rosenstein, MD, MBA
Healthcare Consultant
San Francisco, California
*Improving Physician Communication
    Efficiency: Wants, Needs, and Strategies*

Chapter 8

Elizabeth Scala, MSN, MBA, RN
Owner
Nursing from Within
Jarrettsville, Maryland
*Nursing From Within: Your Inner Guidance
    System to Whole-Person Self-Care*

Dev Raheja, MS, CSP
President/Consultant
Patient System Safety
Laurel, Maryland
*Safety of Nurses Improves Patient Safety
    and Quality*

Chapter 9

Rebecca Volpe, PhD
Assistant Professor of Humanities
    and Director
Clinical Ethics Consultation Service
Milton S. Hershey Medical Center
Penn State College of Medicine
Hershey, Pennsylvania
*If It Looks Like a Duck, Swims Like a Duck,
    and Quacks Like a Duck, Then It's
    Probably a Communication Breakdown*

James Murphy
Independent Consultant
Chief Learning Officer
Management 3000
Lynn, Massachusetts
*Some Insights Regarding Organizational
    Culture Change Efforts*

Chapter 10

Suzanne Gordon
Journalist, Patient Safety Expert
San Francisco Bay Area, California
*Team Intelligence and the Pursuit
    of Genuine Teamwork*

Chapter 11

Diana M. Crowell, RN, PhD, NEA-BC
Nursing Education and Leadership Consultant
Kittery, Maine
Animal Spirits and Complexity

Chapter 12

Stephanie Frederick, RN, Med
Owner
Integrated Health
Tucson, Arizona
*Finding the Courage and Recognizing Our
    Worth!*

Leilani Schweitzer, BA
Patient Liaison
Stanford University Hospitals & Clinics
Reno, Nevada
An Education I Wouldn't Wish on Anyone

Chapter 13

Keith Carlson, RN, BSN, NC-BC
Board Certified Nurse Coach
Santa Fe, New Mexico
Nurses, Culture, and Communication

Paul Gross, MD
Assistant Professor
Albert Einstein College of Medicine
Bronx, New York
We're Not So Very Different

Chapter 14

Brittney Wilson, BSN, RN
Clinical Informatics Nurse and Professional
    Blogger
TheNerdyNurse.com
Villa Rica, Georgia
*Avoiding Potential Pitfalls With Electronic
    Medical Records and Social Media*

Erica MacDonald, RN, BSN, MSN
Nurse Educator
Henry, Tennessee
Healthcare Transparency and Online
*   Diligence for Nurses*

Chapter 15

Rose O. Sherman, EdD, RN, NEA-BC,
**   FAAN**
Professor and Director, Nursing Leadership
    Institute
Christine E. Lynn College of Nursing
Florida Atlantic University
Boca Raton, Florida
How to Build a Sense of Community in
*   Your Workplace*

Nance Goldstein, PhD, ACC
Industrial Economist
Working Wisely Group
Resident Scholar
Brandeis University, WSRC
Cambridge, Massachusetts
Engaging Millennial Nurses in a VUCA
*   World: How Every Nurse Leader Can Help*

Debra Bailey, PhD, RN, FNP, CDE
Director of Health Sciences, DNP
    Program Director, Associate Professor
    of Nursing
Colorado Mesa University
Grand Junction, Colorado

Erin Bailey, DNP, RN, FNP-C
Assistant Director SON, Assistant
    Professor
Stephen F. Austin State University
Nacogdoches, Texas

Suzanne L. Bailey, PMHCNS-BC, CNE
Associate Professor of Nursing
University of Evansville
Evansville, Indiana

Shari Cherney, RN, BScN, MHSc
Professor
George Brown College
Toronto, Ontario
Canada

Kelly Coffin, RN, MSN, CCRN
Assistant Professor of Nursing
Colorado Mesa University
Grand Junction, Colorado

Michelle A. Connell, RN, BScN, MEd
Centennial George Brown Collaborative
    Nursing Degree Program Coordinator
Centennial College
Toronto, Ontario
Canada

Susan Estes, RN, MSN
Clinical Associate Professor
Georgia Baptist College of Nursing of
    Mercer University
Atlanta, Georgia

Abimbola Farinde, PharmD, MS
Clinical Pharmacist Specialist
Clear Lake Regional Medical Center
Webster, Texas

Mark J. Fisher, PhD, RN
Assistant Professor
University of Oklahoma College of Nursing
Oklahoma City, Oklahoma

Judith Joy, PhD, RN
Associate Professor, Nursing and Public
    Health
Colby-Sawyer College
New London, New Hampshire

Mary Lou Kaney, MSN, RN
Assistant Professor
St. Ambrose University
Davenport, Iowa

Cheryl Kent, MS, RN, CNE
Assistant Chair and Faculty, Department
    of Nursing
Northwestern Oklahoma State University
Enid, Oklahoma

Brenda S. Lessen, PhD, RN
Assistant Professor of Nursing
Illinois Wesleyan University
Bloomington, Illinois

Jane Lucht, MS, RN
Associate Professor
Edgewood College
Madison, Wisconsin

M. Star Mahara, RN, BSN, MSN
Associate Professor
Thompson Rivers University
Kamloops, British Columbia
Canada

Gwen N. McCartney, MSN, BSN, RN, BSBA, CNE
Nursing Instructor
Union University
Jackson, Tennessee

Nancy McLoone, RN, MS, CPNP
Assistant Professor
Minnesota State University
Pediatric Nurse Practitioner
Mankato Clinic
Mankato, Minnesota

Robert J. Meadus, BVocEd, BN, MSc(N), PhD, RN
Associate Professor; Associate Dean pro tempore Undergraduate Programs
Memorial University School of Nursing
St. John's, Newfoundland and Labrador
Canada

Mary E. Minton, PhD, RN, CNS
Associate Professor of Nursing
South Dakota State University
Rapid City, South Dakota

Jessica L Naber, RN, PhD
Assistant Professor
Murray State University
Murray, Kentucky

Christine Pilon-Kacir, PhD, RN
Professor of Nursing
Winona State University
Rochester, Minnesota

Yvette M. Rose, RN, DNPc
Assistant Professor of Nursing
Olivet Nazarene University
Bourbonnais, Illinois

Nancy Simpson, MSN, RN-BC, CNE
Associate Professor, Nursing
University of New England
Portland, Maine

Charlene M. Smith, DNS, MSEd, WHNP, RN-BC, CNE
Professor
St. John Fisher College
Rochester, New York

Landa Terblanche, PhD
Associate Professor
Trinity Western University
Langley, British Columbia
Canada

Patricia Thompson, PhD, RN
Professor
Winona State University-Rochester
Rochester, Minnesota

Mary Ann Troiano, DNP
Associate Professor
Monmouth University
West Long Branch, New Jersey

Marian Underdahl, MSN, RN, CNE
Nursing Instructor
North Idaho College
Coeur d'Alene, Idaho

Wendy Wheeler, RN, MN
Instructor
Red Deer College
Red Deer, Alberta
Canada

Krista Wilkins, RN, PhD
Assistant Professor
University of New Brunswick
Fredericton, New Brunswick
Canada

ACKNOWLEDGMENTS

I am grateful for the many people who in various ways helped me to conceive and write *Successful Nurse Communication*.

Thank you to my dear son and friend, Curran B. Russell; my mother, Dorothy Boynton; and my wonderful inner circle of friends: Diane Brandon, Cher and Ronnie Brigham, Marilynn and Steve Carter, Cheryl Greenfield, Jiahong Juda, Jorinda Margolis and Paul and Nate Fitzpatrick, Colleen Poirier, and Paula Schwach. I appreciated your listening and encouragement more than you know. I am also grateful for help along the way from Judy Ringer, Don Russell, Nancy and Richard Schmid, Peter Smith, and Deb Van Winkle.

Thank you to the people who have helped to keep me healthy in body, mind, and soul: Robbin Anderson, Marilynn Carter, Pamela Henry, Honore LaFlamme, Pam Neff Montembeau, and all my Zumba buddies at Jubilation!

Thank you to all of the professionals who wrote inspiring essays for the "Confident Voices" features. Your varied and expert perspectives provide valuable insight, experience, and knowledge to this book and make this project truly collaborative.

Thank you to the team at F.A. Davis, including Tom Ciavarella, Echo Gerhart, and Julia Curcio for believing in and encouraging the mission of this book and for bringing it into being. And thank you to the nurse reviewers who provided constructive feedback across the chapters.

Finally, editors deserve special mention because they bring a much needed skill set to the table and, when combined with a commitment to the ideals of a book, become trusted co-pilots in the process. Thank you Amy Reeve for editing this book and Bonnie Kerrick, RN, BSN, for editing my first book, *Confident Voices*, which was indeed a stepping stone to *Successful Nurse Communication*.

TABLE OF CONTENTS

PART IV: SUCCESSFUL NURSE COMMUNICATION IN ACTION   173

Welcome to *Successful Nurse Communication*! Wherever your career takes you (or you take it), your communication skills as a nurse professional will play an integral role in your ability to provide safe and quality care, be a positive influence on your workplace teams and culture, and sustain your enthusiasm for ongoing learning. *Successful Nurse Communication* aims to empower you to be a responsible team player, respectful change agent, and full partner in the work of improving patient safety in healthcare systems, while at the same time encouraging you to create a career path that is exhilarating and in alignment with the hopes and expectations you have as nursing student and/or nurse who is continuing his or her education.

Effective communication skills, from an intellectual perspective, are fairly simple and straightforward. However, from the perspective of human behavior, they are vastly more complicated. To learn to communicate effectively, professional growth must interface with personal growth in core areas of emotional intelligence, such as awareness of self and others, motivation, and self-esteem, that inform assertiveness and respectful listening, which in turn contribute to team development and healthy workplace cultures.

Successful Nurse Communication takes a unique approach to building essential communication skills because of its emphasis on developing the interrelated emotional intelligence necessary to speak assertively and listen respectfully in the high-stakes, high-pressure environments in which professional nurses work every day. This text presents a strong foundation of research and weaves in real-world examples and case studies designed to engage students and promote personal reflection and group discussion. As well, each chapter contains two additional features: The "Confident Voices" features comprise inspiring and varied perspectives from clinicians, consultants, and patient advocate experts in the field on topics that complement and in some cases elaborate on the chapter content, whereas the "Consultant Commentary" features provide more informal glimpses into the authors' experiences as a nurse and nurse consultant that reinforce the learning in the book.

Successful Nurse Communication strives to promote the six aims of high-quality healthcare that care be safe, effective, patient-centered, timely, efficient, and equitable defined by the Institute of Medicine (IOM; 2001) in its report, *Crossing the Quality Chasm*. The book also sets out to develop competencies recommended by the IOM's subsequent report, *Healthcare Professions Education* (National Research Council, 2003): that nurses must provide patient-centered care, work in interdisciplinary teams, employ evidence-based practice, apply quality improvement practices, and utilize informatics. These aims and competencies for nursing education are incorporated in the following goal and objectives for this text:

Goal

To increase nurses' ability to practice safe, effective, patient-centered, timely, efficient, and equitable care through effective communication and collaboration

Objectives

- To increase nurses' effectiveness with patient, family, and interprofessional communication
- To increase awareness and promote discussion among nurses, students, and colleagues regarding the interrelatedness of effective communication with patient care, self-care, and the healthiness of workplace cultures, teams, and systems
- To provide a resource for teachers, individuals, facilitators, and leaders that builds nurses' abilities to practice effective communication skills, develop professional behaviors, and become positive change agents in today's complex healthcare environments

- To further the commitment to these ideals, students will gain an appreciation for how effective communication is integral to the Quality and Safety Education (QSEN) Institute's competencies (Cronenwett et al., 2007) to continuously improve care and to promote every nurse's ability to pursue a rewarding career as a competent, compassionate, and respected healthcare professional.

Online Resources

Electronic resources for instructors and students are available on Davis Plus:

For Students

- Davis Digital Version (enhanced ebook)
- Multipart interactive case studies
- Videos demonstrating interpersonal communication

For Instructors

- Davis Digital Version (enhanced ebook)
- A chapter-by-chapter Instructors Guide which includes:
  - Chapter-At-A-Glance
  - Exercises for Experiential Learning
  - Answer Key for Case Study Questions
  - Commentary for Reviewing Reflection Questions
  - PowerPoints (1 presentation per chapter)
- Test bank

Visit Davis*Plus*.com and use the instructions on the inside cover of your book to start using these helpful resources. (Instructors: your F.A. Davis Sales Representative will provide you with access to all instructor and student resources.)

Congratulations for taking part in this dynamic journey toward the mastery of communication and collaboration that is so vital for every nurse and the patients and families we serve. Let's begin!

References

Cronenwett, L., Sherwood, G., Barnsteiner, J., Disch, J., Johnson, J., Mitchell, P., ... Warren, J. (2007). Quality and safety education for nurses. *Nursing Outlook, 55*(3), 122–131.

Institute of Medicine. (2001). *Crossing the quality chasm: A new health system for the 21st century.* Washington DC: National Academies Press.

National Research Council. (2003). *Health professions education: A bridge to quality.* Washington, DC: National Academies Press.

Developing Successful Nurse Communication

Part I is devoted to creating a vision of successful nurse communication and to building a foundation of emotional intelligence. Also emphasized are the skills associated with effective and respectful assertiveness and listening, including giving and receiving constructive feedback. In addition to providing the more traditional basics of communication models, styles, and processes, this text promotes a behavioral approach to teaching and practicing the material, which is highlighted in Part I. In these beginning chapters, students will start to appreciate how complicated and essential effective communication is in meeting the goal of providing safe, effective, patient-centered, timely, efficient, and equitable care.

CHAPTER 1

Communication and Behavior

Communication is a critical component of the nurse's mission to assess, plan, implement, and document care. It is present in each collaboration of nursing and allied health colleagues, physicians, and administrators and in every interaction with patients and their families. Ensuring that the right information is obtained and passed along to the right person at the right time in the right way can mean the difference between life and death.

On the surface, speaking up and listening seem like such simple tasks that students may wonder why it is necessary to read a book about or take a course on these skills. However, effective communication is surprisingly complex. There are compelling and interrelated reasons for making the study of communication a priority for nursing students and for engaging them in a career-long commitment to becoming effective communicators. First, there are infinite variables that affect communication—most notably, human behavior, which can be messy, emotionally charged, imperfect, and unpredictable. Studying human behavior is not an easy task, especially in an industry with a strong emphasis on research and evidence. Second, the complexity of communication in healthcare and its relationship to human behavior have not been sufficiently valued and, as a result, continue to be at the root of serious and persistent problems in healthcare.

Successful nursing requires effective communication, which takes a professional commitment to develop and demands skills very different from those required to start an intravenous line or memorize anatomy. Nurses must develop an emotional maturity that will enable them to hold difficult conversations, respect a wide range of diversity, manage conflict, and collaborate effectively. This chapter introduces a vision of successful nurse communication and describes why a behavioral approach is necessary for learning and practicing it. Next, students are introduced to the communication process and explore several important models and common styles. Learning these fundamentals is necessary to mastering the effective communication skills imperative in providing safe care, creating positive workplaces, and sustaining rewarding, long-term careers as nurse professionals.

A VISION OF SUCCESSFUL NURSE COMMUNICATION

Nurses make up the biggest workforce in healthcare and are present at every imaginable juncture. They are the backbone of direct care—from admission to discharge, from health and wellness to death and dying, in every specialty area, 24 hours a day. They serve people of all ages from all cultures and socioeconomic statuses. They work in clinics, hospitals, and long-term care facilities as well as at insurance companies and for attorneys. They are self-employed entrepreneurs and senior-level leaders. Beyond their ubiquitous presence, nurses are perceived by the public to be the most ethical and honest profession (Swift, 2013). This combination of presence and trust puts nurses in a position to act as positive change agents along the entire spectrum of healthcare delivery. It is an exciting and honorable place to be, and one that demands the best that every nurse has to offer all the time. Every nurse must be accountable for developing his or her best self and bringing this best self to every interaction with patients, colleagues, teams, and organizations. **Effective communication** is an essential component every step of the way.

Effective communication can be found in all of the following examples:

- The nursing student reminding a classmate to wash her hands after a central line dressing change
- The newly graduated nurse asking for help and support from her supervisor in assisting with a procedure she has not done before
- The maternity nurse patiently explaining for the third time what a new and anxious mother can do to help her infant breastfeed
- The long-term care nurse calling an elderly patient's daughter in the middle of the night to tell her that her mother is showing signs of actively dying
- The operating room nurse telling the surgeon who has been verbally abusive that he expects to be treated respectfully
- The medical-surgical nurse letting her colleagues know that she is not going to participate in gossip about another nurse
- The emergency room nurse sitting quietly with a man whose wife just passed away and is waiting for family to arrive
- The intensive care nurse answering a plea from his supervisor to stay for an additional shift by saying, "No, I am too emotionally and physically exhausted to work safely"
- The nurse preceptor sharing constructive feedback with a new nurse about her need to do a better job with sterile technique, and the new nurse listening to the feedback and acknowledging an opportunity to develop the skill while holding her head up high

The nurses in these scenarios are confident and assertive. They approach difficult conversations and emotionally charged situations with compassion, an openness to learn, and effective communication skills. They respect themselves and others, and they are able to provide safe patient care under stressful circumstances. They engage in conflict while embracing opportunities to learn from other viewpoints. They set limits for themselves, at the same time respecting the needs and limits of others. They collaborate respectfully with and provide care for people who represent the full range of human diversity. They enjoy their work overall, are enthusiastic about ongoing learning, and bring positive energy into their work environments. They honor their own health and well-being while acting as patient advocates. All of these elements encapsulate successful nurse communication.

A BEHAVIORAL APPROACH TO COMMUNICATION

Successful nurse communication cannot occur without understanding and factoring in human behavior. Human behavior has a strong impact on the expression of thoughts, feelings, opinions, and ideas. While communication is the exchange of messages, behavior affects *how* messages are exchanged. Trying to study or teach one without the other does not fully appreciate either and contributes to oversimplified or superficial solutions not adequate for producing effective communication skills.

To excel at communicating effectively, individuals must be willing to engage in deeper learning about themselves and others. As suggested earlier, part of the reason this skill set has not been effectively developed in healthcare professionals, including nurses, is that so much of traditional learning is intellectual. Mastering clinical skills, such as giving an injection or inserting a catheter, is done first in a simulation laboratory and then eventually on real patients, with supervision. It involves an understanding and recall of the procedure as well as coordination, dexterity, and familiarity with equipment. In mastering communication, understanding and recall are still important, but practicing requires self-reflection, discussion, personal growth, and social learning—a skill set that is difficult to hone, yet vital.

Self-reflection, discussion, personal growth, and social learning are aspects of communication that cross over into the knowledge, skills, and attitudes (KSAs) that nurses must manifest in behavior with patients, families, and colleagues. The pre-licensure KSAs developed by the Quality and Safety Education for Nurses (QSEN) Institute (Cronenwett et al., 2013) provide curriculum guidelines for preparing nursing students to continuously improve the quality and safety of the healthcare systems in which they will work. QSEN delineates KSAs for the six competencies developed by the Institute of Medicine (IOM): patient-centered care, teamwork and collaboration, evidence-based practice, quality improvement, safety, and informatics (National Research Council, 2003). Looking at these guidelines with communication and behavior in mind reveals KSAs in which both are included, even if not obviously stated:

- "Provide patient-centered care with sensitivity and respect for the diversity of human experience" (Cronenwett et al., 2007, p. 123) is a skill for the competency of patient-centered care that will be acquired as nurses become aware of and respect what is important to others. Communication comes into play because nurses must ask questions respectfully in order to assess clinical status and to understand a patient's needs, preferences, and concerns. Recognizing nonverbal language, reading social cues, and honoring the perspectives of others requires understanding of human behavior.

- "Acknowledge own potential to contribute to effective team functioning" (p. 125) is an attitude listed under the competency of teamwork and collaboration. Recognizing the relationship between communication and behavior is important because nurses who have self-awareness and awareness of others, and who understand team development, will be able to use their strengths effectively in collaborative efforts and in opportunities for growth.

- "Recognize that nursing and other health professions students are parts of systems of care and care processes that affect outcomes for patients and families" (p. 127) is an area of knowledge listed in the competency for quality improvement. From a behavior perspective, to gain this knowledge, nurses must have a respectful sense of self and others in order to actively and collaboratively participate in the larger worlds of their units and organizations, practice effective communication, and become positive change agents.

These and many more of the KSAs recommended by QSEN call on nurses to develop effective communication and recognize the role that human behavior plays in the process, including challenging emotional growth, risk taking, and overcoming fears and insecurities. This kind of work is not easy, especially because the very nature of healthcare keeps nurses in a reactionary mode of attending to almost constant clinical priorities. Time for managing conflict, giving and receiving constructive feedback, and developing positive relationships among diverse populations is limited. As students gain an appreciation for the challenging work involved in becoming effective communicators, they will be better prepared to be positive change agents and meet the goals recommended by QSEN and IOM.

Now that students have a vision of what successful nurse communication looks like and its relationship to behavior, they are ready to examine the fundamentals of the communication process, beginning with styles and types.

Confident Voices

Renee Pontbriand, RN, ADN ADPM
Nursing Supervisor, and Visiting Nurse

Modeling Good Behavior

As the weekend supervisor in a long-term care and rehabilitation facility, a typical day for me starts at 6:30 a.m., going from unit to unit to communicate with both the nurses and 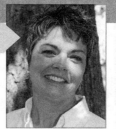 licensed nursing assistants (LNAs) about how their night went, what residents are having issues that need to be addressed that day, and staffing issues or concerns. As a nursing supervisor, my job duties include upholding facility policy and procedures as they pertain to the care of the residents and patients. Nowhere in my job description does it identify "how" this is to be done. Granted, most people would say that it is knowing those policies and procedures like the back of your hand and implementing them as needed. That is not enough. A successful nurse knows that it starts with communication, mutual respect, and sincerity for his or her coworkers, who include all of the people that keep a facility running smoothly—housekeeping, dietary, laundry, and maintenance.

I make it a point to say "good morning" to all of my coworkers and ancillary staff. I ask them how things are going at any given time during the day. As a result, these staff members do not hesitate to help out the nursing staff, whether it is cleaning up

Continued

Confident Voices—cont'd

an overflowing toilet, retrieving durable medical equipment (DME) out of the storage area, or washing personal laundry in the event a resident does not have adequate clothing for the day. Ancillary staff members keep an extra set of eyes and ears on patients as they walk through the units performing their own job duties.

Communication not only is about expressing your ideas and expectations clearly regarding how something is supposed to be done but also is about being a good listener and really caring about the people you work with. It is about lending a hand when the unit is staff-challenged and working side by side with your LNAs to identify issues before they become emergencies for both patients and staff. I consider my facility one big home; in fact, many of us spend more time here than we do in our actual homes. This is also our residents' permanent home, and the responsibility of all of us to promote respect for, concern for, and a commitment to the people we care for.

I have also learned that, as nurses, we are always role models for each other; whether we make good decisions or bad, someone is always watching and learning how to be an effective professional—or not. Good decisions may come in the form of calling a doctor at the early signs of a resident health issue and not leaving it for the next shift to deal with, not leaving orders to be followed up on during the next shift if possible, and placing a blank nursing note in a chart when there is no more room on the page to write on.

On a daily basis, we are mentors for everyone we come in contact with on the job. I believe we have the ability to demonstrate patience, compassion, and understanding in any healthcare environment—a winning situation for ourselves, our coworkers, and, most important, our residents.

Biography
Renee Pontbriand, RN, ADN, ADPM, is the weekend nursing supervisor in a rehabilitation and long-term care facility and a per diem RN in home health. She is a member of the Worldwide Leaders in Healthcare, and her professional interests include geriatrics, geropsychology, home health, and nurse mentorship.

COMMUNICATION STYLES AND TYPES

Individuals typically use one of four styles of communication: aggressive, passive-aggressive, passive, and assertive. Each reflects a sense of one's own values and needs at that particular instance as well as life experiences and behavioral patterns that have developed over time. Nurses should focus on understanding what these communication styles look like in practice settings as well as consider what styles they tend to use most.

Individuals with an aggressive communication style are more concerned with their own needs than those of others. Such people can be abusive toward others and may or may not be aware of their impact. Characteristic behaviors of an aggressive style of communication include the following:

- Dominating group discussions
- Frequently interrupting others
- Invading others' personal space
- Using verbal or nonverbal language to humiliate, judge, or otherwise disrespect others
- Ignoring or discounting others' perspectives
- Speaking in an angry and often loud voice
- Physically assaulting or throwing objects at others

Passive-aggressive communication is indirectly aggressive but can still be abusive. Individuals who practice this style believe that their needs are just as or more valuable than others', but they do not overtly express aggression. Characteristic behaviors include the following:

- Gossiping about others behind their back
- Using body or nonverbal language that is incongruent with verbal language
- Telling jokes that have discriminatory themes or using sarcasm
- Sabotaging or resisting change
- Excluding others from a group activity

Individuals who practice a passive style of communication seem to believe that their opinions, values, or needs are not as important as those of others. The ideas and concerns of these individuals are rarely, if ever, presented, many times resulting in a loss of respect and esteem for themselves and in the eyes of others. Characteristic behaviors include the following:

- Apologizing frequently
- Discounting one's own opinions
- Fidgeting and other nervous body language
- Giving up or letting others occupy their personal space
- Using excessive language
- Assuming participation in a group would not be helpful or wanted

Assertive communication is a style in which individuals recognize that their needs are important but that so are the needs of others. Characteristics of an assertive style include the following:

- Respecting others' perspectives even when disagreeing
- Respecting one's own and others' personal space
- Speaking confidently and clearly
- Using respectful verbal and nonverbal language
- Contributing to group efforts and listening to others

Assertive communication is the most respectful and professional style and is recommended by this author. However, it can be challenging to be an assertive communicator, particularly in an aggressive culture where there is little to no reciprocity of respect. Assertive communication does not come naturally for many nurses and requires a significant commitment to develop. Assertiveness will be discussed in more depth in Chapter 4.

Consultant Commentary

I have been a practicing RN for more than 25 years and, for about a decade now, a consultant specializing in communication and collaboration for healthcare professionals. I earned my graduate degree in Organization and Management, with a focus on group dynamics, emotional intelligence, and organizational behavior. Developing my own assertiveness has been a part of my journey along the way.

In my master's program, we did a lot of work in small groups and were required to be fully participating team members. As a more introverted person, and formerly a bit passive, I gained insights about my own tendencies to hold back and became aware of how uncomfortable I felt being in a leadership role, even though I had great ideas. Eventually, I came to realize that the groups I was part of wanted and needed my perspective in order to do the best teamwork possible. I also discovered leadership qualities I was not aware I had. Gradually, I learned to take more risks and share my ideas, and I found it helpful when my classmates asked for my views and listened.

As I continue practicing as an RN, I also continue to study, practice, and write about communication in healthcare. Working in home health, occupational health, and long-term care venues, I have become acutely aware of how ineffective communication skills and related behaviors contribute to poor outcomes. They are pervasive factors in all sorts of issues, including medical errors, burnout, poor patient experiences, work-related injuries, and workplace abuse. Awareness of these factors continues to be reinforced from my vantage point as a consultant as well as a practicing RN.

As a consultant, I enjoy facilitating interactive workshops on communication and collaboration with nurses. In teaching assertive communication to individuals who have varied tendencies toward passive, aggressive, and passive-aggressive communication and behaviors, the goal is always the same—to develop assertive communication—but the learning for each individual is different. In general, people who are aggressive must learn to listen and respect others, people who are passive must learn to respect and speak up for themselves and others, and people who are passive-aggressive must learn to do both. When one person becomes a better listener and another becomes more assertive in speaking up, collaboration becomes a productive process in which we contribute, learn, problem-solve, and co-create. Everyone gains from the collective knowledge, experience, and wisdom that become available.

Beyond the four styles, there are two types of communication: verbal and nonverbal. Verbal communication refers to the actual words used in conveying a message; some words may mean different things to different people for reasons including cultural influences, age, education, and native language. **Nonverbal communication**, which typically represents 80% to 90% of what is being communicated, involves tone, facial expression, stance, gestures, intonation, and pace. Both verbal and nonverbal communication types are part of any face-to-face interaction.

Miscommunication occurs when the receiver's understanding of the message differs from what the sender was intending. (Read about using validation and clarification skills to avoid miscommunication in Chapter 3.) When messages are perceived as honest, that is often because the nonverbal language is consistent with the verbal message. Not surprisingly, if a verbal message is truthful, the body's expression naturally emits the same message. When individuals are saying something that they do not really mean or that is a partial or complete lie, their nonverbal language may give them away. If a colleague says, "I'd be happy to help," while walking away, rolling her eyes, and sighing heavily, she is implying that her words are not sincere. This is an example of a mixed message because her words are saying one thing and her behavior and body language another. Of course, body language can be misleading. Maybe she has reasons for walking away and rolling her eyes that have nothing to do with her offer for help. Nurses must be mindful of aligning their verbal communication and nonverbal communication.

MODELS OF COMMUNICATION

Numerous models have evolved to portray the communication process with varying degrees or layers of complicating factors. Going back to the 1940s, early models, such as one developed by mathematician and engineer Claude Shannon, portray communication as a linear one-way process in which the sender transmits a message to the receiver. Shannon described the process with seven basic elements: sender, encode, message, receiver, decode, channel, and noise (Shannon and Weaver, 1949). His linear process is illustrated in Figure 1.1, in which the *sender encodes* a *message* and sends it to the *receiver* who interprets or *decodes* it. The *channel* represents the path of transmission, such as phone, e-mail, or face-to-face communication. The *noise* refers to any interference or distortion, such as a background noise, a choppy reception, or a speaker who mumbles.

In 1970, a transactional model of communication was developed by scholars, including Dean Barnlund (1970), who proposed that communication is a reciprocal process of feedback and messages between individuals in an effort to create common meaning. Barnlund's model, illustrated in Figure 1.2, depicts a more complicated process of communication. Factors influencing messages being sent back and forth include feedback, noise, and context, such as the mood of the communicators, the social setting, and both separate and shared experiences.

In *Communication for Nurses: How to Prevent Harmful Events and Promote Patient Safety*, Pamela McHugh Schuster and Linda Nykolyn (2010) introduce a more complicated **transformational model of communication** that focuses on desired outcomes of the process and links to patient safety. Their model, illustrated in Figure 1.3, uses concentric circles to portray how the more basic process of communication takes place through layers of *context, risk factors,* and *patient-safe communication strategies* to influence the desired outcome of *transformation,* where actual change takes place. The transformational model depicts how complicated communication is and helps to explain why miscommunication or communication failures are so prevalent in nurse practice areas involving patient safety, abuse in the workplace, and patient experience, all of which are explored in later chapters.

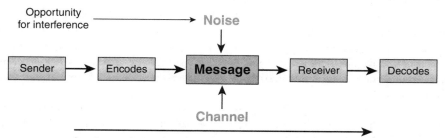

Figure 1-1 Linear model of communication. (From Schuster, P. M., and Nykolyn, L. *Communication for nurses: How to prevent harmful events and promote patient safety.* Philadelphia: F. A. Davis Company, 2010, p. 14. Reprinted with permission.)

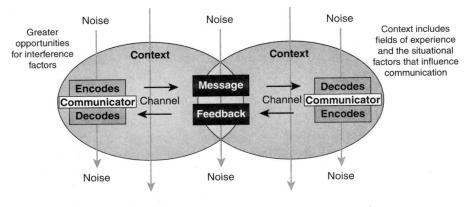

Figure 1-2 Transactional model of communication. (From Schuster, P. M., and Nykolyn, L. *Communication for nurses: How to prevent harmful events and promote patient safety.* Philadelphia: F. A. Davis Company, 2010, p. 16. Reprinted with permission.)

VARIABLES THAT AFFECT COMMUNICATION

When considering factors such as workload, interruptions, varying levels of trust, and gender and ethnic differences, the variables that influence communication seem endless. As mentioned previously, the most basic definition of communication involves the sender and the receiver of a message and the message itself. For example, a nurse reports concerns about changes in a patient's condition to a physician. The sender of the message is the nurse, the receiver is the physician, and the message is the patient's condition. A simple and straightforward exchange of information between two colleagues has occurred.

But much of the time, the healthcare environment is not so simple and straightforward. Consider the following scenario: A nurse calls a doctor and reports an increase in a patient's blood pressure, and the physician orders a new test as well as changes in medication. This communication seems fairly routine, but there are a number of elements in play behind the scene that affect the sender, the receiver, and the message. The physician on call does not know this patient. The patient's blood pressure has been fluctuating up and down during the day, and this latest spike may not necessarily be an unexpected or new pattern. The nurse from the previous shift was in a hurry and forgot to mention to the nurse coming on duty that the patient's regular doctor is aware of the fluctuation. Unaware of this, the nurse currently on duty considers calling the physician at home, but she is hesitant because it is 3:00 a.m. and this particular doctor is known for his quick temper. The nurse's efforts to check the medical record for details of the previous shifts are slowed by trouble logging into the hospital's network. And just as the nurse decides it is best to call the doctor at home, another patient falls out of bed. How quickly this simple communication became far more complicated!

The purpose of this book is to integrate the complexity illustrated by Schuster and Nykolyn's model into a practical strategy for learning communication that is fluid in the real world of human behaviors. Such a behavioral approach will prepare individuals to become more aware of and develop healthy responses to infinite variables (e.g., cultural differences, history of poor

(Continued on p. 14)

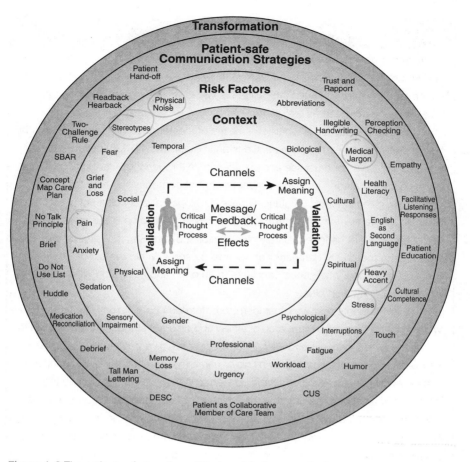

Figure 1-3 The patient-safe transformational model of communication. (From Schuster, P. M., and Nykolyn, L. *Communication for nurses: How to prevent harmful events and promote patient safety.* Philadelphia: F. A. Davis Company, 2010, p. 17. Reprinted with permission.)

Confident Voices

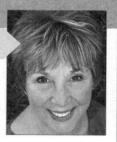

Candace Campbell, DNP, RN, CNL
Assistant Professor of Nursing and Health Science

As Guests in Our Patients' Home

"All the world's a stage," said Shakespeare in *As You Like It* (1997, Act 2, Scene 7), "and all the men and women merely players. They have their exits and their entrances, and one man in his time plays many parts." As members of the human family, we nurses are blessed to be privy to some of the best and worst stages in a total stranger's life. How can we create the safest and most positive workplaces?

Continued

Confident Voices—cont'd

An important element in your development toward becoming an effective nurse and communicator involves what Daniel Goleman (1995) dubbed *emotional intelligence* (see Chapter 2). Goleman builds his whole theory around the idea that we must see with our heart as well as our eyes.

In my experience, this is where the realms of theater and nursing run parallel. In his seminal text, *An Actor Prepares*, Constantin Stanislavski (1936) devotes two volumes to how an actor must see and experience life through the eyes of the character he portrays. An actor's worldview must be that of compassion, even to the villain, who might, given other circumstances, have developed a totally different personality. After all, we are all members of the human family. Imperfection is our cross to bear, so to speak. All of us face trials and temptations, posits Stanislavsky, so who are we to judge the crusty demeanor of another person? Within the scope of nursing practice, emotional intelligence translates to an open and accepting worldview and a safe and caring workplace.

I tell my students that we must learn to enter each patient room as though we were crossing the proscenium arch of a new and different stage, and we must learn to intuit the healthcare experience by the clues we are given. When we imagine ourselves in the place of the patient or as his or her family member, our eyes are opened in a new way to unspoken needs and concerns. We do well to understand the psychology of disenfranchisement theory, which suggests that there are three drivers applicable to the patient experience: alienation, cynicism, and perceived victimization. Feelings of disenfranchisement may make even the most brave among us behave like a frightened, cornered animal, so be prepared. Consider this, take a breath, and then calm yourself.

As soon as you set foot in the room, you absorb information: How many people are there? Are there any safety issues, such as equipment lines dangling low? Liquid or obstacles on the floor? Intravenous site infiltrated? Catheter tubing kinked? Dressing clean and dry? Room too hot or cold? Simultaneously, you notice the less obvious: What seems to be the atmosphere? What does the patient's or visitors' tone and mannerisms of speech, facial expressions, and body language tell us? If there are other professional personnel in the room, you notice how the patient is involved in that experience: Does she seem interested? Frightened? Pleased?

Next, while you inwardly list the tasks at hand and their order of importance, you seek to present yourself in a professional manner, yet kind and caring. How best to accomplish this? Approach the patient as though you were a guest in his or her home. This simple inverse of perception will go far to establish an atmosphere of respect, which your patient will (usually) immediately perceive. Consider that your patient's only real estate at the moment is the furnishings in this room. Furthermore, the patient usually would rather be somewhere—anywhere—else than in this bed, having to face the consequences of a health problem that requires the intervention of a team of strangers. The patient has been stripped of worldly possessions and made to fit an institutional mold.

Here are 10 steps to establishing effective patient communication:

1. First, LISTEN.
2. Unless there is an emergency, address the immediate voiced concerns.
3. State clearly and calmly the nature of your business in that room, and stop.
4. LISTEN.
5. Address any and all remaining concerns of patient and family.
6. Renegotiate elements of treatment related to time schedules, pain medication, and so on, as possible.
7. By asking open-ended questions, take a few moments to learn how the patient is coping with the disease, hospitalization, and treatments.
8. LISTEN.
9. Restate what you heard.
10. State what you might do to take a step in solving a dilemma, or, depending on the situation, take the time to sit with the patient and LISTEN some more.

As a nurse, you are a healthcare representative—a navigator, educator, advocate, and guardian of hope. When you view your work with the open worldview that all humankind is one family, you see with the heart. When you do that, as Antoine de Saint-Exupery (1943, p. X) says, you learn that "what is essential is invisible to the eye."

Of course, not everyone will embrace this philosophy. There will be toxic environments where you will need to evaluate when your usefulness there is expended. Despite such setbacks, when you see with your heart, your experiences will usually match your expectations that life is beautiful and that nursing is a call to embrace all of humanity.

References

Goleman, D. (1995). *Emotional intelligence: Why it can matter more than IQ.* New York: Bantam Books.

de Saint-Exupery, A. (1943). *The little prince* (K. Woods, Trans.). New York: Harcourt Brace and Company.

Shakespeare, W. (1997.) *As you like it*. B. A. Mowat & P. Werstine (Eds.). New York: Washington Square Press. (Original work published 1623.)

Stanislavski, C. (1936). *An actor prepares* (E. Reynolds Hapgood, Trans.). New York: Theatre Arts Books.

Continued

communication, interruptions, or fatigue) that are part of the communication process as it occurs moment to moment in real life. Using a behavioral approach combined with mastering speaking up and listening, nurses will be prepared to navigate a wide range of challenges skillfully and compassionately.

CASE STUDY

Sheila is a student nurse on a medical-surgical clinical rotation in a busy teaching hospital. Although she has many years of experience as a licensed practical nurse (LPN) in a long-term care facility, this is her first experience in an acute setting. Sheila's patient is Mr. Strombowski, a 45-year-old man on his second postoperative day after an emergency laparoscopic appendectomy with a suspected perforation. The reporting nurse tells Sheila that his temperature yesterday was as high as 100.6°F and that he received two hydrocodone-acetaminophen tablets at 2:00 a.m. with good effect. He's on intravenous antibiotics, and cultures are pending. The surgeon was in to see him at 6:00 a.m., and there were no new orders. Sheila has had telephone conversations with this surgeon, and he has a reputation for being abrupt. He is scheduled to be in surgery all day. At 9:00 a.m., the patient's temperature is 100.5°F, and he's complaining of abdominal pain. He had two hydrocodone-acetaminophen at 8:00 a.m. There are parameters to call the physician for a temperature higher than 101°F. At 9:30 a.m., Sheila checks the patient's temperature again, and it is 100.6°F; he also reports that "the pills didn't help" his pain. Sheila talks with the covering nurse and her instructor. Although the covering nurse says that she should only call the surgeon if Mr. Strombowski's temperature goes any higher, her instructor agrees that a call to the surgeon now is appropriate.

Discussion Questions

1. How would Sheila deliver her message to the surgeon using an assertive style? Using a passive style?

2. How might the surgeon's reputation for abrupt behavior be influencing the covering nurse's decision to call only if the patient's temperature increases?

3. What concerns might Sheila have about making the phone call?

4. Create a list of possible circumstances that might influence the surgeon's response.

SUMMARY

Communication is closely related to human behavior and affected by skill, practice, and experience as well as culture (ethnic and organizational), gender, emotional intelligence, personality, and stress. Effective and respectful communication is an imperative goal for nurses, but it is not simple to master. In the next three chapters, respectful listening and assertiveness will be explored in more depth, and emotional intelligence will be introduced. At this point, students should have a deepening sense of appreciation for the importance and complexity of respectful communication among the healthcare team and with patients and families.

Reflection Questions

1. Consider a clinical experience in which you were responsible for teaching a patient about a medication. Beyond the intellectual aspects of teaching, were there behavioral factors, for either you or your patient, that may have influenced communication?

2. Review the list of examples of nurses practicing effective communication earlier in this chapter. Pick two or three that might be challenging for you. Why do you think they would be, and what might help you to increase your comfort level in similar situations?

3. Review the four common styles of communication. Can you think of any examples of situations in which you have practiced any or all of them? Do you believe you have a particular style that you use most frequently?

References

Barnlund, D. C. (1970). A transactional model of communication. In K. K. Sereno & C. D. Mortensen (Eds.), *Foundations of communication theory* (pp. 82–102). New York: Harper and Row.

Cronenwett, L., Sherwood, G., Barnsteiner, J., Disch, J., Johnson, J., Mitchell, P., . . . Warren, J. (2007). Quality and safety education for nurses. *Nursing Outlook, 55*(3), 122–131.

National Research Council. (2003). *Health professions education: A bridge to quality.* Washington, DC: National Academies Press.

Schuster, P. M., and Nykolyn, L. (2010). *Communication for nurses: How to prevent harmful events and promote patient safety.* Philadelphia: F. A. Davis Company.

Shannon, C. E., and Weaver, W. (1949). *The mathematical theory of communication.* Champaign, IL: University of Illinois Press.

Swift, A. (2013, December 16). Honesty and ethics rating of clergy slides to new low: Nurses again top list; lobbyists are worst. *Gallup Politics.* Retrieved from www.gallup.com/poll/166298/honesty-ethics-rating-clergy-slides-new-low.aspx.

CHAPTER 2

Emotional Intelligence

- Understand the importance of developing emotional intelligence in order to practice effective communication and collaboration
- Identify three models of emotional intelligence
- Describe the competencies of emotional intelligence according to Goleman's model and their connection to communication and collaboration
- Understand the importance of optimizing respectful relationships at work when possible while conducting professional behavior at all times

KEY TERMS

- Emotional intelligence
- Self-awareness
- Self-regulation
- Motivation
- Empathy
- Social skills

Communication and collaboration are inseparable from human behavior; consequently, they are informed in part by emotions. Developing one's emotional self is therefore integral to developing respectful listening skills and assertiveness. How individuals feel and act on or express their feelings at any given moment involves such variables as life experience, wants, needs, limitations, and skills. In the late 1990s, the term *emotional intelligence* was coined to describe the awareness, processing, and management of the vast variety of feelings that humans experience. Nurses will be better prepared to practice effective communication if they understand the impact of emotions on themselves and others. This knowledge base will enhance sensitivity toward others and contribute to nurses' ability to provide patient-centered care, embrace diversity, manage conflict, and be collaborative members of their healthcare teams. In recent years, nursing research literature has covered studies supporting the importance of emotional intelligence in leadership (Cummings, Hayduk, & Estabrooks, 2005; Molter, 2001; Vitello-Cicciu, 2002), exploring the relationship of emotional intelligence with occupational stress and health in nurses (Augusto Landa, López-Zafra, Berrios Martos, & Aguilar-Luzón, 2008), and identifying connections of emotional intelligence to coping, social support, and mental health in nursing students (Montes-Berges & Augusto, 2007).

This chapter introduces students to the field of emotional intelligence (also known as EQ and EI) by first describing three primary models and then exploring the one developed by psychologist Daniel Goleman in greater depth. Students will examine its five competencies while focusing on their relevance to communication and collaboration in nursing practice.

MODELS OF EMOTIONAL INTELLIGENCE

There are three well-known conceptual models of **emotional intelligence**: ability, personality, and mixed. The ability-based model was introduced by psychologists Peter Salovey and John D. Mayer (1990) and considers emotions as resources for navigating one's social environment. Their theory evolved to consist of four abilities: identifying emotions of self and others, using emotions to facilitate reasoning, understanding emotions in self and others, and managing emotions in self and emotional situations (Mayer, Salovey, & Caruso, 2000).

The personality-based model, developed by psychologist Reuven Bar-On (1997), uses an inventory of attributes that are self-reported and categorized by five constructs: intrapersonal (self-awareness and self-expression), interpersonal (social awareness and interpersonal relationships), stress management (emotional management and regulation), adaptability (change management), and general mood (self-motivation).

The mixed model was introduced by Daniel Goleman, who brought the term *emotional intelligence* into the popular culture with his groundbreaking, best-selling book, *Emotional Intelligence: Why It Can Matter More Than IQ* (1995). His theory combines abilities with personality traits. In his subsequent book, *Working With Emotional Intelligence*, he elaborates on two competencies of emotional intelligence: personal, which includes self-awareness, self-regulation, and motivation; and social, which includes empathy and social skills (Goleman, 1998).

Among these models, there is significant overlap in the personality traits, behaviors, and competencies used to describe how emotional intelligence is defined and measured. Further discussion of the larger realm of emotional intelligence is outside the scope of this text. However, Goleman's model will be explored in more depth next to highlight the value of a behavioral approach to communication and collaboration in the context of nursing practice.

Confident Voices

Erika Hunter, MEd
Knowledge Manager

The Benefits of Naming Emotions
Putting feelings into words makes sadness and anger less intense, U.S. brain researchers said [recently], in a finding that explains why talking to a therapist—or even a sympathetic bartender—often makes people feel better. They said talking about negative feelings activates a part of the brain responsible for impulse control. (Wolpert, 2007)

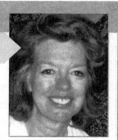

As health professionals, we spend much of our time focused on others—responding to their needs, considering their futures, and formulating plans for them. Helping people places demands on our attention and energies. We mediate situations that are life and death. While we keep our professional selves focused outwardly, our

Continued

Confident Voices—cont'd

inward self is also taking it in, absorbing through our senses everything we see, hear, smell, think, and feel. We collect information and react internally throughout the day. Sometimes what we see and hear is very difficult. So how do we keep communication with ourselves and others sustainable?

We work in circumstances that most people do not. There are day-to-day explicit standards on the job and implied expectations about our personal lives. While maintaining professional distance from patients, yet interacting intensely with them, we are expected, and often expect ourselves, to pick up from wherever we were before coming to work as though the day's events do not affect us.

What, then, happens to those experiences we had? How do those experiences get processed and integrated? In our professional role, we forgo our personal responses; in our lives, we have freedom (and the responsibility) to acknowledge our opinions, judgments, and emotions—in other words, to be known.

Having good boundaries is part of most workplace expectations, which is why recognizing and owning our emotional truth is so important. Some caregivers choose to focus more on their clients' lives than their own. For example, I knew one couple, both of whom were therapists, engaged in an abusive marriage. He occasionally beat her up, and she did not want to end the marriage. For 5 years, they both went to their joint office space looking wonderfully professional, helping others, and fulfilling obligations, after which they went home to tolerate their lives until clients showed up the next day.

Were they effective as clinicians? Yes, they seemed to be. Were they intelligent? Yes, very. Were they hero and heroine to their clients? Yes, they had a very busy practice, each with a good reputation. However, outside the professional role, they were dysfunctional, cruel, and irresponsible. Were they able to talk honestly about their emotions? No. Eventually both were treated for addiction—a disease strongly related to holding onto appearances.

Emotions drive us and hold us back. To be a balanced professional, we must be in a relationship with our feelings. Most of us do not refine our emotional vocabulary, using generalities instead of specifics. (For example, saying "I'm upset" is too general. It can mean anything.) Research has shown that in naming our feelings, we free ourselves of some of the intensity of carrying them.

Naming the five basic feelings—anger, sorrow, gladness, fear, and shame (or mad, sad, glad, scared, and ashamed)—is an easy and effective way to express and let go of carrying responses. The shortest way to express our truth about something is to see which of these is involved: Am I angry? Sad? Happy? Scared? We usually have multiple emotional ingredients combining to create something we call "upset."

For example, if a little boy, badly injured by an adult, is brought into clinic, we feel *upset*. In order to name and let go of the emotion, we must privately acknowledge:

Confident Voices—cont'd

"I am angry that this adult harmed this child. I am sad for this child and scared about his future. I am relieved and glad that the neighbor brought him in."

We can take just 1 minute, whether in the break room or driving home, to acknowledge to ourselves or share with a friend, family, or colleague the truth of our day. We are vulnerable, we are affected, no matter how wonderfully contained we are at work. In being mirrored back, we are validated, loved, and filled back up. The onus of appearing perfect fades away.

Emotions are energetic products—the mix of brain and physical response neurotransmitters, cortisol and thoughts—pushing us to do something. We have choices about how we handle our reactions, from talking to holding on, from losing control to freezing. In recognizing and using "I feel . . ." basics, we can clear out our day emotionally and be more aware of how to support our clients and colleagues.

Reference

Wolpert, S. (2007, June 7). Putting feelings into words produces therapeutic effects in the brain: UCLA neuroimaging study supports ancient Buddhist teachings. *UCLA Newsroom.* Retrieved from newsroom.ucla.edu/releases/Putting-Feelings-Into-Words-Produces-8047.

Biography

Therapist and writer Erika Hunter, MEd, believes that many people lack an emotional vocabulary. To support them, she has written *The Little Book of BIG Emotions: How Five Feelings Affect Everything You Do (and Don't Do)* (2004, Hazelden) that outlines how emotions can be powerful agents for change.

EMOTIONAL INTELLIGENCE IN NURSING

Goleman's (1998) model could serve as a description of competencies necessary for successful nurse communication or, more broadly, positive attributes that all healthcare professionals should aspire to. These competencies require effective and respectful communication, encourage proper professional behavior, and result in better teamwork. Here, the competencies of Goleman's model, personal and social, are correlated specifically to nursing to solidify their importance.

Personal Competence

Self-Awareness

Self-awareness is about understanding one's feelings at any given moment and being in touch with both present causes and past experiences that are contributing to that emotional state. Nurses who are self-aware are able to discern feelings such as frustration, anger, or excitement that relate to their home or social life from those that arise from experiences at work. They know when they are exhausted or overwhelmed, stay grounded in the present, seek appropriate support, and practice respectful expression of wants and needs. Self-awareness and respect for one's emotions is crucial for setting healthy limits, asking for and accepting help when needed, and offering help when available. A nurse who requests training and seeks out resources for more information most likely has an accurate self-awareness of her needs, wants, skills, and readiness to learn. This is in sharp contrast to the nurse who is emotionally and/or physically exhausted and lacking awareness of and/or respect for the limitations stress places on her ability to provide safe, compassionate safe care and to ensure her own well-being.

In addition, having self-awareness contributes to self-confidence. As nurses learn to respect their own abilities and knowledge, they will be more comfortable when faced with something they do not know; rather than see it as an indication of inadequacy, they will recognize it as a learning opportunity. Such nurses can admit when they do not know something, bring ideas to their team, accept constructive feedback, and sustain positive self-worth in stressful situations and toxic workplace cultures.

Consultant Commentary

I was in my ninth hour of a second 12-hour shift. A combative patient was in the bathroom with a nurses' assistant while I was outside the room trying to quickly measure out 0.5 cc of topical Ativan. The other nurses' assistant was on break, and the third had called in sick. The medication in gel form sticks a little to the syringe, and it can be tricky to get the full dose without pushing too far on the plunger. I was trying to concentrate. I had not taken a meal or rest break and was worried about the patient and the aide, and, of course, I did not want to make a medication error. A visitor approached me at the medicine cart and asked me for the code to get out of the locked unit. Even though I raised a finger to signal to wait, she asked again for the code to get out. Meanwhile, the phone was ringing, another patient's call light went on, and I could hear the yelling escalating in the bathroom several yards away.

Inside, I was furious, but I put down the syringe and calmly told her the code. In that moment, I was aware that my anger and frustration were resulting from the current stressful situation combined with a long shift with limited staff. The visitor left, and I administered the medication, successfully diffusing the combative patient. No one was hurt, and I did not make a medication error. I was relieved about that, but I knew that either could have happened all too easily.

My self-awareness about the intensity of my feelings and all of the contributing stressors (staffing shortages, length of shift, time management, and lack of breaks) is part of my emotional intelligence. It is a personal barometer that helps me set limits and ask for help, both of which are necessary for safe care and my own health. Also, as I learn to respect my own barometer, I can appreciate and respect others. A different nurse might not have been so tired or stressed in that moment or may have been more stressed and expressed anger inappropriately. (According to other nurses, I had replaced a nurse who had been terminated for losing his temper at a family member.) Later that week, I had a conversation with my manager about all of the stressors I was facing; she suggested a few ideas that I promised to try. Over the next few months, I was more proactive about taking meal breaks and asking the supervisor to help cover my breaks when short-staffed, but the sick calls were chronic and the supervisor frequently unavailable, and so I eventually left the position.

Emotional intelligence by itself does not solve problems such as staffing or time management, but it is an essential part of the equation. As more nurses are able to recognize and respect their own and others' limits, they will be contributing to long-term, meaningful solutions.

Self-Regulation

Self-regulation refers to how a person responds to various situations and requires ownership of several elements. Feeling angry and thinking about acting aggressively are natural, but nurses who self-regulate are able to acknowledge thoughts and feelings first, and then channel their actions in appropriate and healthy directions. Nurses who are able to self-regulate can control aggressive or passive behaviors and remain calm under stress. Being aware of impending loss of self-control provides a nurse with a moment to stop to take a deep breath and count to ten to avoid an inappropriate response in a highly charged situation.

To master self-regulation, nurses must learn to be transparent when appropriate. Being open and honest about feelings, beliefs, and actions in various roles and circumstances can be important, especially when needing to take ownership of mistakes and misunderstandings and in developing a healthy approach to conflict. However, some privacy is valuable in maintaining professional and personal boundaries.

Adaptability is another element of self-regulation. Nurses must learn to be comfortable, or mostly comfortable, with the constantly changing landscape of delivering healthcare. Change should be seen through a lens of new opportunities. Nurses must learn to how to express their own wants and needs as they respond to change. Nurses who develop expertise at setting limits based on awareness of needs will ultimately be more flexible and able to compromise.

Motivation

Motivation to fulfill unmet needs and desires is a driving force of human behavior. By learning about and understanding their own motivation, nurses can make personal and professional decisions that help them grow. (A nurse's role in motivational interviewing will be discussed in Chapter 6.) Nurses' needs often take a back seat in day-to-day work environments, where they must focus the needs of patients, families, doctors, administrators, and other healthcare professionals. Whether by nature, through life experience, or through professional expectations, nurses may become more adept at identifying their patients' needs than their own. To some extent, this is inherent in the work. However, being able to recognize their own needs and understand the motivation behind them is extremely important to safe care, patient satisfaction, and long, healthy careers.

All nursing students become familiar at some point in their coursework with Abraham Maslow's (1999) hierarchy of needs, which has evolved over the years to include eight levels: physiological, safety and security, belonging and love, esteem, cognitive, aesthetic, self-actualization, and self-transcendence. Nurses learn about the hierarchy of needs in relation to patient care, but it is as relevant to nurses as it is to patients. A nurse asking a peer to administer pain medication to a patient while she takes a meal break is an example of assertive behavior that is motivated by needs such as hunger, stress, and belonging.

Motivation is also necessary for achievement, such as working to maintain a high standard of professionalism or participating in lifelong learning and ongoing career development. The key is to set goals that are challenging yet attainable and to engage in risk-taking behavior that is aligned with a genuine sense of self. Getting into and through nursing school is a great testimonial to nurses' capacity for this aspect of personal competence.

Finally, taking initiative and being optimistic are more ways to practice self-motivation. Nurses must take action to influence care, culture, and career in positive ways by actively engaging in finding resources, providing input, and solving problems. They must believe that their actions and input will be respected; make a difference in patient, team, and organizational outcomes; and contribute to rewarding careers.

When nurses become skilled in all areas of personal competence, it will result in more assertive behavior and more effective communication.

Confident Voices

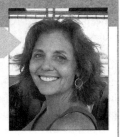

Jorinda Margolis, LICSW
Social Worker

How Compassion and Mindfulness Can Decrease Suffering
So, in this life of ours stuff happens. Not the stuff we take time and dreaming to plan and look forward to, but rather the painful stuff.

We get sick, we miss planes, relationships end, jobs are lost (as are car keys and important papers). We make mistakes, and accidents happen. Despite our best plans and intentions, in our mortal human lives, we experience pain. Perhaps emotionally, perhaps physically, and more often than not, we suffer.

Often, pain comes into our lives because of events and outcomes outside of our control; yet it is our minds that determine how much we suffer. Our perceptions, beliefs, and thoughts create a story about our pain. Often, our minds tell stories about ourselves. Stories of how we somehow caused our pain through ineptitude, stupidity, or poor planning. We fault ourselves for many of the events that just happen.

Perhaps we do this because we want to believe that we are fully in charge of our lives and that with a magic balance of assertiveness and carefulness we could be pain free.

Using this framework of pain versus suffering, we can turn to the vast power of our minds to sort out the pain from the suffering—not to let ourselves off the hook for circumstances over which we have little control, but to focus our minds and grow our empowerment through self-compassion.

In my clinical practice, I often ask my clients if they would ever be as hard on others as they are on themselves. After 20-plus years as a therapist, no one has ever replied "yes"! As we grow our self-talk to include acceptance that life's circumstances are not always agreeable and to show ourselves some compassion, knowing that life's difficulties are not the result of our inadequacies, we will surely decrease our suffering.

We can also grow our acceptance in conversations with others. Accepting that disagreement is a normal part of human interaction can vastly decrease our suffering as well as the suffering of the person we are in conversation with. As we bring some acceptance to mind, we immediately decrease our suffering. In this calmer space,

Confident Voices—cont'd

we may also find an opportunity to hear something new, perhaps a unique perspective that might lead to a further decrease in suffering for ourselves—a self-narrative that includes appreciation and validation for all that we have accomplished in service to a kind and gentler world, for the opportunities we have taken to bring forward compassion and to ease the suffering of others. This is a mindful and compassionate inner dialogue that does not lack humility or demand perfection. It is our recognition that we are, as the saying goes, "only human" and likely quite fine humans at that.

Biography

Jorinda Margolis, MSW, received a Graduate Fellowship from Boston University School of Social Work. She has practiced in a variety of settings, including schools, an inpatient child and adolescent psychiatric unit, state child protective services, a community mental health facility, and, most recently, group and individual private practice settings. She has advanced postgraduate training in trauma, dialectical behavior therapy, EMDR, integrative wellness, and attachment issues arising from adoption and trauma. She currently has a private practice in Exeter, New Hampshire, teaches continuing education, and provides clinical consultation to individuals and organizations.

Social Competence

Empathy

Empathy is defined as the ability to understand another person's circumstances, point of view, thoughts, and feelings. When experiencing empathy, a person is able to understand someone else's internal experiences (Salters-Pedneault, 2014). It is in essence how humans demonstrate caring and respect for others, and for nurses, it is important in establishing a therapeutic relationship with patients and professional relationships with colleagues. Nurses must be able to read a limitless range of emotional cues from patients, families, and peers. Close attention paid to verbal and nonverbal language increases the information available for assessing and understanding what is important to others and helps in identifying underlying issues and relevant solutions. Nurses who develop the capacity to have and show empathy are more likely to treat patients with dignity and compassion. This is a vital part of the bridge between the science and the art of nursing practice. Nurse scholar Theresa Wiseman (1996) describes empathy as a combination of four attributes: taking the perspective of another person, not judging others, recognizing emotion in other people, and being able to communicate that recognition. Students who wish to get a better idea about what empathy looks and feels like in healthcare are encouraged to check out Cleveland Clinic's (2013) YouTube video, "Empathy: The Human Connection to Patient Care."

Social Skills

Social skills involve the ability of a person to observe the environment around him or her and to use what is learned to influence communication and collaboration. This skill set is very important because all nurses will come up against conflict, work with diverse colleagues and care for a diverse population, and be put into leadership situations. The inherent qualities that individuals bring to or develop in their job inform their workplace relationships, which in turn influence teamwork and organizational culture and patient outcomes. It makes sense that positive or at least respectful relationships will make the workplace more pleasant and have an impact on retention of staff as well as quality and safety of care, whereas negative relationships will do the opposite. Having respectful relationships is a part of being professional. However, although positive relationships can enhance collaboration, it would be unrealistic to insist on them as a prerequisite for behavior. The challenge, then, is to encourage nurses to build and nurture positive relationships, with the caveat that such relationships do not always need to be in place to provide safe and quality care. In other words, nurses have to rely on each other even when there is conflict and tension. By behaving respectfully at all times, nurses can minimize the negative impact of unhealthy professional relationships and workplace cultures. The importance of healthy relationships will take on even more meaning when students get to Part III, in which organizational culture, teams, and complex adaptive systems are explored.

CASE STUDY

It is 2:30 p.m. on the medical-surgical floor, and day shift RNs Jasmine, Jeffrey, and Rose are finishing up their documentation and getting ready to give report to the oncoming shift. The nurse manager approaches and asks, "Will one of you stay until 7:00 p.m.? Wanda's son came home from school sick, and she can't get a sitter until later."

Jasmine rolls her eyes and lets out a huge sigh. She wants to get home early and get ready for a weekend trip to visit a friend. She answers, "I guess I could, but I still haven't finished all my charting. I'm already behind, but if you really want me to, I'll stay." Inside, she is feeling annoyed with and resentful of her peer who is unable to come in on time.

Jeffrey does not feel very tired and probably could handle a few more hours, but he does not want to. He has long thought that Wanda uses her daughter as an excuse to get out of work at times. He tells the nurse manager he is not going to cover for her but stays silent as to why.

Rose takes a deep breath. She is on her sixth day in a row and is looking forward to 3 days off with her family. She does not want to stay either but feels she can compromise. "I'm really tired, but I'm willing to stay. However, I'll need an assignment I can handle easily while tired and that won't put myself or patients in any danger."

Discussion Questions

1. How would you describe Jasmine's response with respect to Goleman's competencies of emotional intelligence? What suggestions do you have for her to develop greater emotional intelligence?

2. How would you describe Jeffrey's response with respect to Goleman's competencies of emotional intelligence? What suggestions do you have for him to develop greater emotional intelligence?

3. Describe how Rose's response differed from Jasmine's and Jeffrey's. In what ways did she demonstrate highly developed emotional intelligence?

4. Consider how the nurse manager might respond to each of these nurses. What conversations and outcomes can you envision?

SUMMARY

Emotional intelligence offers a framework for developing awareness and skills that contribute to important professional growth and reveal insights into the complexity of human behavior. In any model of emotional intelligence, there are elements that involve understanding and managing one's own emotions as well as those of others. As students develop awareness about their emotions and align their behaviors using honest self-reflection, patience, and respect for others, there is enormous opportunity for improving quality of care and sustaining rewarding careers in nursing. The skills that allow for learning and practicing personal competencies of emotional intelligence are interrelated with developing assertiveness, and those that involve social competencies are interrelated with becoming a respectful listener. These are the roots to building workplace cultures of mutual respect in which collaboration will arise out of contributions from every member.

Reflection Questions

1. Review Goleman's emotional intelligence competencies discussed in this chapter and choose one that you'd like to develop as part of your plan for a meaningful and rewarding career as a nurse. Consider how you will go about it, what support you might need, and whom you know that could be a resource.

2. What led you to choose a career in nursing? Do you hope to have any of your needs from Maslow's hierarchy met as a nurse professional? If so, reflect on what they are and why they might be important to you.

3. Consider a patient you have cared for during a clinical rotation. Were you able to feel and show empathy for that person? Describe how you did, or, if you did not, how you could in the future.

4. Do you think you can work respectfully with all of your classmates? If there are exceptions, what might hold you back, and what ideas do you have for addressing any conflicts?

References

Augusto Landa, J. M., López-Zafra, E., Berrios Martos, M. P., & Aguilar-Luzón, M. d. C. (2008). The relationship between emotional intelligence, occupational stress and health in nurses: A questionnaire survey. *International Journal Nursing Studies, 45*(6), 888–901.

Bar-On, R. (1997). *The Bar-On emotional quotient inventory (EQ-i): Technical manual.* Toronto, Canada: Multi-Health Systems.

Cleveland Clinic. (2013). Empathy: The human connection to patient care [video]. Retrieved from youtube.com/watch?v=cDDWvj_q-o8&feature=kp.

Cummings, G., Hayduk, L., & Estabrooks, C. (2005). Mitigating the impact of hospital restructuring on nurses: The responsibility of emotionally intelligent leadership. *Nursing Research, 54*(1), 2–12.

Goleman, D. (1995). *Emotional intelligence: Why it can matter more than IQ.* New York: Bantam Books.

Goleman, D. (1998). *Working with emotional intelligence.* New York: Bantam Books.

Maslow, A. (1999). *Toward a psychology of being* (3rd ed.). New York: Wiley & Sons. (Original work published 1986.)

Mayer, J. D., Salovey, P., & Caruso, D. (2000). Models of emotional intelligence. In R. J. Sternberg (Ed.), *Handbook of intelligence* (pp. 396–420). New York: Cambridge University Press.

Molter, N. C. (2001). *Emotion and emotional intelligence in nursing leadership* (Doctoral dissertation). Santa Barbara, CA: Fielding Graduate Institute.

Montes-Berges, B., & Augusto, J. M. (2007). Exploring the relationship between perceived emotional intelligence, coping, social support and mental health in nursing students. *Journal of Psychiatric and Mental Health Nursing, 14*(2), 163–171.

Salovey, P., & Mayer, J. D. (1990). Emotional intelligence. *Imagination, Cognition, and Personality, 9*(3), 185–211.

Salters-Pedneault, K. (2014). What is empathy? A definition of empathy. Retrieved from bpd.about.com/od/glossary/g/empathy.htm.

Wiseman, T. (1996). A concept analysis of empathy. *Journal of Advanced Nursing, 23*(6), 1162–1167.

Vitello-Cicciu, J. M. (2002). Exploring emotional intelligence: Implications for nursing leaders. *Journal of Nursing Administration, 32*(4), 203–210.

CHAPTER 3

Respectful and Effective Listening

LEARNING OBJECTIVES

- Explain why listening is a critical skill for nurse professionals
- Explain the difference between listening to assess and listening to understand
- Identify the three common styles and the five stages of listening
- Describe steps necessary to becoming a respectful and effective listener
- Explain how the GRRRR model for listening can be used to receive critical information about a patient
- Increase ability to effectively receive feedback

KEY TERMS

- Reflective listening
- Passive listening
- Competitive listening
- True curiosity
- Perspective-taking
- Validation

Respectful and effective listening is the receiving part of the communication loop. *Respectful* refers to the listener's mindset toward the speaker, and *effective* refers to the message being received and understood as intended. Respectful and effective listening is often more complicated than meets the eye. In this chapter, critical areas and styles of listening are explored along with techniques that help optimize the listening part of the communication process. Strategies that focus on becoming a respectful listener are also discussed. There are endless opportunities for nurses and students to practice, develop, and role-model listening, and a variety of personal and professional challenges go along with developing the skill.

WHY LISTENING IS VITAL

Communication is occurring in one way or another at all times. The more effective the listening, the more likely the message being sent will be understood and the more effective the overall communication will be. In nursing, there are three critical areas in which listening is a paramount responsibility.

The first is in making clinical assessments. Nurses use listening skills when taking patient histories and patients' subjective complaints. Close attention must be paid to a patient's verbal and nonverbal messages, and clarification must be sought when necessary to ensure that the most accurate information possible is obtained. The nurse's clinical role is to ask questions to develop an appropriate care plan (e.g., What's your normal bowel pattern? How much alcohol do you consume? What spiritual or religious preferences are important to you?). Careful listening is also required when nurses auscultate a patient's blood pressure or bowel sounds, participate in a patient handoff, and receive doctors' orders. As patients move from the emergency room to the intensive care unit to the medical-surgical floor and finally home, nurses play an important role in making sure important information (e.g., laboratory results, treatment instructions, current medication regimens, new and old allergies, patient and family concerns) are passed on to and understood by the next healthcare team and/or the patient and caregivers. Nurses must make sure that they are accurately translating and transcribing doctors' orders. Effective listening in the middle of a noisy environment, especially when dealing with a physician or colleague who is in a hurry or displaying disruptive behavior, is a vital skill.

Second, effective listening is critical when attempting to understand patients and others. In listening to understand a patient's concerns, needs, or perspective, nurses are listening less as clinical practitioners and more as fellow human beings who want to gain a sense of what matters to the patient. This also applies to communication with patients' families as well as all members of the healthcare team. In the day-to-day work of busy healthcare professionals, it is easy to forget this aspect of listening. Listening to understand conveys compassion and creates opportunities to engage others, and it is the responsibility of every team player. Consider the following scenario: A nurse is assessing the smoking history of a male patient who has, unknown to her, lost a family member to lung cancer. There may be cues that the patient has more to say but that he may not feel comfortable or may think the nurse is too busy or not interested. For instance, does the patient hesitate when answering or start to say something and then stop? Does his facial expression change, or does he seem more anxious when answering this question than others? It is very important for nurses to take the time to explore and acknowledge what is going on with a patient. When nurses are busy, they may be reluctant to offer feedback, build trust, and probe for further information. However, the nurse who puts her pen down or takes her focus off the computer screen and offers her attention is likely to learn more. She also gives the patient the sense of being cared for. Going back to the scenario just given, let's assume the nurse considers the patient's cues and says, "I get the sense that you are very worried about your smoking habits. Would you share a little more?" While taking the time to listen is indeed more time consuming, in this case the nurse's recommendations about smoking cessation are more likely to be heard, understood, and considered. These moments—when nurses see and treat patients as people with concerns and fears—are privileged intersections for practitioners and patients. They demonstrate the "care" in healthcare and the art of nursing.

The third area in which effective listening is key is in managing conflict. Although many nurses would prefer to avoid conflict, the reality is that conflict is unavoidable. Conflict may arise because of differences in expertise, education, available information, and time pressure; varying personality types or characteristics in the workforce or patient population may also bring about conflict. Many conflicts have the potential for increased knowledge as well as collaborative and creative problem-solving, but without good listening practices, conflicts often end up unresolved. Lingering resentment or counterproductive power struggles may interfere with collaboration. In such cases, learning opportunities are lost, teamwork suffers, and patient care is compromised.

Even though it is critical, finding the time and space for listening can seem insurmountable. There are three things nurses can do that will have a positive impact on raising awareness about the value of listening and ensuring that there is time allotted for doing it. First, practice it. People in general appreciate being heard, and practicing listening will raise awareness about the value it brings. Second, pay attention to successes associated with listening and share these stories with other nurses: "I'm glad I took a few extra minutes with Mrs. Brown before her surgery this morning. I wouldn't have known about the allergic reaction she had to penicillin." Third, be assertive about the need for more time to listen. This might involve a request to a colleague or unit manager, such as, "Could you hang an IV antibiotic for Mrs. Smith? I need 15 more minutes with Mr. Jones before he goes home. He's finally relaxed with me and has a lot of questions about his medications."

LISTENING STYLES

Complementary to knowing *when* to listen is recognizing the different styles of listening. There is a lot of literature and nomenclature that describe listening using overlapping definitions and similar language. This book focuses on three common styles of listening: reflective, passive, and competitive.

Reflective Listening

Reflective listening, sometimes referred to as *active listening*, is a model developed by organizational theorist Dalmar Fisher (1993) in his book, *Communication in Organizations*. It is a core skill used in mental health counseling and is associated with patient- or client-centered communication. In essence, reflective listening requires a very conscious and intentional focus on the person speaking. The primary objectives are to demonstrate empathy for the speaker and to ensure that his or her message is understood. It can be especially useful when someone is stressed or vulnerable, such as a patient who is anxious about being hospitalized or has just received bad news about a biopsy. Reflective listening requires concentration, caring, and commitment and is accomplished by following two steps.

The first step is to make listening to the speaker the priority. This means not thinking about other tasks, people, or worries and ensuring a conducive environment (i.e., with privacy and without any or at least minimal interruptions). This is very difficult because nurses often have an endless list of urgent and constantly shifting priorities and frequent interruptions. True reflective listening can take more time, especially when initially developing the skill. Yet patients and staff who feel heard are much more likely to ask questions, follow recommendations, share concerns, and feel less anxious—all of which contribute to better outcomes.

The second step is to validate (described in greater detail later in this chapter) and demonstrate empathy with occasional nodding and utterances such as "hmm" or "ahh" to show interest, understanding, and concern. Empathy is also portrayed verbally by paraphrasing key points the speaker is making and clarifying when necessary. For instance, a patient might say, "I know I should be eating healthier meals, but every time I try, something stressful happens and I start binging on junk foods again." The reflective listener's response would sound something like, "It sounds like healthy eating is really important to you, and stressful situations make it harder. Is that right?" Such a response will help the speaker feel listened to and validated and also give her the chance to clarify or add more to the story. In this case, there is the opportunity to discover underlying stressors that may be going on for this patient and possibly illuminate a different priority. Without this deeper, more comprehensive listening process, the nurse could document that a nutritional assessment was completed but would miss an opportunity to obtain important information. Spending more time listening will help target the most critical problem, saving resources in the long run.

Passive Listening

Passive listening, also called *attentive listening*, encourages a mutual approach in which all participants are paying attention to each other. There is an assumption of understanding and an expectation that opportunities to talk will be balanced with opportunities to listen. Reflective listening may weave in and out of such conversations if there are misunderstandings or if the emotional tone changes, indicating that one person needs to be heard more than another. Imagine a nurse who is complaining to a colleague about being assigned yet again a difficult patient. If they are both engaged in passive listening, the colleague might say, "I hear your concerns about working with Mrs. Fitzpatrick again today. She is very demanding and rude at times. But I already have three patients who I don't know at all and would really like to keep the other two I'm familiar with." This offers the other nurse the opportunity to speak up and offer a compromise: "I can understand that. What if I take on one of your patients who you don't know?"

Consultant Commentary

During interactive workshops on communication skills, I find that nurses already know how to listen effectively and respectfully, why it is important, and what makes it hard. In fact, I start the workshop by asking, "What does respectful listening look like?" The language varies from group to group, but the essential ingredients are usually provided (e.g., honest, nonjudgmental, validating). The next question I ask is, "Why is respectful listening important in nursing?" Most group members know the answers to this, too, and will offer answers such as that it helps improve safety, helps patients feel cared for, and helps us to learn. And when I ask them what makes it hard, they are eager to share experiences, including lack of time, interruptions, lack of staff, and conflict—all very real stressors that I and most other nurses can relate to. It may sound silly to ask questions that I know they know the answers to, but the process is very important. By listening to them and validating their ideas, I am role-modeling effective listening, engaging them in the work, and building trust. I am also creating a safe environment in which all voices are heard and valued.

However, this knowledge only covers the intellectual aspects of listening, and we fail to improve the skill when we use training methods that only address these aspects. In my workshop, after we've gone over the intellectual aspects, the behavioral learning takes place as I coach nurses in practicing the skill. We put their knowledge to the test by practicing activities involving challenging scenarios provided by the group. Seeing a different perspective when in an emotionally charged conflict is extremely difficult. Having the participants' trust and respect allows me to coach them through difficult conversations that require self-reflection and present ownership challenges. I often get feedback that nurses do enjoy and learn from the brainstorming and practice sessions. I believe that behavioral in addition to intellectual learning is needed to become more effective communicators, and that's what I try to teach in my workshops.

Competitive Listening

Competitive listening, also called *combative listening*, is an approach that focuses on disagreeing or arguing with the speaker and moving the conversation in a direction the listener wants it to go in. A competitive listener is constantly thinking about a response to challenge the speaker rather than really listening to what he or she is saying. This is a passive-aggressive or aggressive way of using the conversation to express the listener's voice or to discount the speaker rather than trying to understand the message or the receiver. A person who is a competitive listener may have a more urgent need to be heard or control the conversation and/or lack the assertiveness skills to show ownership. Knowing about this style is important so that nurses can identify it in themselves and others. A nurse with this listening style can and should work to develop better listening skills because a patient's ability to learn is questionable during a conversation with a nurse who is a competitive listener.

STAGES OF LISTENING

Beyond the three common styles, listening can be broken down into five stages: hearing, attending, understanding, remembering, and responding (Beebe, Beebe, & Redmond, 2014). Each of these components is subject to multiple influences that affect how the message is received.

Hearing

Hearing, the actual physiological process of listening, requires the ability to hear words or read sign language in order to receive a message. Reading a letter, email, or text from someone is also a form of taking in information from someone else and is included in the hearing component. Reading this book is even a form of hearing because this author is conveying a written message to students. Listening is influenced by factors such as one's ability to hear, read, see, or understand verbal, written, or sign language, including foreign languages, as well as a variety of other factors, including environment, distance, and volume.

Attending

Attending refers to the listener's focus on the verbal and nonverbal expressions of the person speaking. Distractions, disinterest, and strong emotional connection to the message or speaker are examples of variables that may influence the listener's ability to pay attention.

Understanding

Understanding is best accomplished by paraphrasing, clarifying, and avoiding assumptions. The exception is when a basis of understanding has already been established through attentive listening (i.e., with friends or colleagues). The importance of clarifying and validating another's message in order to ensure understanding is underscored by the many variables that affect it.

Remembering

Remembering is an important step in honoring the speaker and using the information. Writing things down, bookmarking pages, and entering data in a computer are familiar ways of remembering information. Given the almost constant influx of new and vital information, nurses should be in the habit of recording important subjective and objective data soon after obtaining them.

Responding

Responding is essential for letting the speaker know he or she has been heard and understood. Nodding, clarifying, and validating are all responses. Without this step, patients and colleagues may feel ignored, even when the listener has been paying attention. For example, a nurse may find it frustrating to delegate a task to a nursing assistant who walks away without any acknowledgement that the message was received. The nurse's assistant may be committed to doing the task, but the nurse would have no way of knowing it.

BECOMING A RESPECTFUL LISTENER

Knowledge of listening styles and stages provides the basis to take active steps in improving listening skills. Following are guidelines for becoming a respectful and effective listener.

Develop True Curiosity

True curiosity is an important foundation for listening respectfully. Questions, often considered to be the hallmark of curiosity, are useful in assessing patients, portraying attentiveness, and clarifying messages. Nurses are taught to use inviting language such as, "Tell me more" or to ask open-ended questions when inquiring about a patient's history, at the same time being careful not to make judgments consciously or subconsciously. These important techniques for obtaining accurate reports and assessments are subtly different from true curiosity. True curiosity arises from a deeper desire to understand and learn more about someone else's interests, concerns, or experiences.

Demonstrating curiosity can aid a nurse in determining the real reason behind a patient's behavior. A patient calling for pain medication before it is due may need a dose adjustment or may have anxieties associated with a history of poorly managed pain. The nurse who is curious about why the patient is calling so soon is more likely to get at the underlying reason. True curiosity can also help nurses establish compassionate relationships with patients in which they are viewed as human beings and not only as patients with symptoms to analyze.

Confident Voices

Briana Pefley, BSN, RN
Charge Nurse

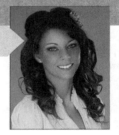

The Spirit of Inquiry, Evidence-Based Practice, and Developing Your Innate Curiosity

The spirit of inquiry, the absolute foundation of evidence-based practice (EBP), is a reasonably simple concept, yet seems to be lacking from the everyday skills set of many healthcare professionals. Where would healthcare be today had no one ever questioned routine practices? Well, I'm personally thankful that someone got around to questioning the use of "tobacco-smoke enemas," which were commonly used to treat headaches and other ailments in the early 1800s. In order for EBP to evolve, influence practice, and ultimately improve patient outcomes, healthcare professionals need to get reacquainted and comfortable with constantly asking questions.

When I think of the spirit of inquiry, I often think of that inquisitive child we've all encountered at some point in our lives. You know, that little boy who always has a

Confident Voices—cont'd

follow-up question for every answer his mother presents him with. Consider the following example:

Mom: "We are going to the grocery store Kenny."
Kenny: "But why, Mommy?"
Mom: "Because we need food to grow big and strong."
Kenny: "But how does food make me big and strong, Mommy?"
Mom: "Because food has vitamins and minerals."
Kenny: "But why do I need 'vi-mins' and 'minrales,' Mommy?
Mom: "Because I said so, Kenny, get in the car."
Kenny: "But why?"

Okay, you get the idea. Children are like little sponges of wonder trying to soak up as much knowledge about the world as possible; they are always asking questions, and they love to push limits. Healthcare professionals could learn a lot from children. Why as we grow older do we stop asking questions and start taking "because I said so" as an answer? I have found that, as adults, we are often so focused on having the right answer that we stop asking questions. Perhaps my personal experience can shed some more light on this subject.

As a relatively novice nurse with only 2 years of professional experience, my colleagues often refer to me as "naïve" or "green" when I question routine policies or practices. As much as I respect and admire my seasoned coworkers, it seems that over time, they've succumbed to "because I said so" as an explanation and have stopped asking questions altogether. In the few instances that I have questioned practices, armed with the latest research, I have been met with skepticism and, often, belittlement. In those cases, it was almost like I was the little boy described earlier, and the policymakers were my mother: "Now, now, honey, leave those decisions to the grown-ups."

When nurses are not actively engaged in their work, they become complacent, and unfortunately this complacency is the crux of the problem: "When a spirit of inquiry—an ongoing curiosity about the best evidence to guide clinical decision-making—and a culture that supports it are lacking, clinicians are unlikely to embrace evidence-based practice" (Melnyk, Fineout-Overholt, Stillwell, & Williamson, 2009, p. 49). So, if healthcare professionals are uncomfortable or unfamiliar with asking questions, and their respective employers do not encourage this curiosity, how will EBP ever evolve?

I escaped this complacency myself thanks to my recent enrollment in an MSN program. My research methods and health policy classes were particularly insightful

Continued

Confident Voices—cont'd

and played a large role in revitalizing my own spirit of inquiry. My professors were actively engaged with us and encouraged students to ask questions of each other, making for spirited discussions and an enhanced learning experience. However, this art of questioning needs to be fostered and encouraged long before graduate school. Here are some tips I wish I had learned earlier in my career:

- **Find EBP mentors.** Seek out professional role models now, such as professors or nurse educators where you plan to work. Networking now will help ensure you are prepared when you are faced with adversity in the real world.
- **Join professional organizations.** Many organizations offer student member prices. They will keep you up to date with the latest EBP initiatives and ways to get involved. Organizations are also a great networking tool.
- **Remember that knowledge is power.** Understand where to find the latest research and interpret it effectively. Your EBP mentors and professional membership can assist with this.
- **Start asking questions again.** Whether in the classroom or at work, start getting comfortable with asking questions again. You should also know whom to go to with questions regarding policies or practices.
- **Choose wisely.** Choose to work in a healthcare organization that encourages employees to get involved with EBP. Typically those with Magnet accreditation or "Transforming Care at the Bedside" initiatives are a good place to start looking.

You have an obligation as a healthcare professional to fight for both your patients and your profession. Your education does not and cannot stop after your degree is earned. Remember why you went into healthcare in the first place: to help people. Lifelong learning is the only way to ensure that "because I said so" does not become a suitable explanation for you and that your patients do not suffer as a result.

References

Melnyk, B. M., Fineout-Overholt, E., Stillwell, S. B., & Williamson, K. M. (2009). Igniting a spirit of inquiry: An essential foundation for evidence-based practice. *American Journal of Nursing, 109*(11), 49–52.

Biography

Briana Pefley, BSN, RN, is a charge nurse pursuing an MSN in Nursing Education and Adult Gerontology with plans to practice as a certified clinical nurse specialist in the acute care setting. She is also a nurse educator with goals to write for publication.

Practice Openness to Other Perspectives

Listening respectfully involves being open to another's viewpoint, which is especially challenging when another person's perspective includes an opposing opinion, particularly on a sensitive topic. Abortion, stem cell research, and unionization are some topics about which people often have strong opinions and may have trouble considering perspectives different from their own. **Perspective-taking**, or being open to other points of view, does not require giving up or even challenging one's own opinion, although there is often a great fear of that. Many conflicts remain unproductively stuck in power struggles because individuals are unable to see other viewpoints and are focused on being heard rather than listening.

A nonthreatening way to practice perspective-taking is to view an optical illusion such as the rabbit/duck image in Figure 3.1. People often see either the duck or the rabbit when first looking at the picture. After they learn that the other image is also present, many readily see both. In addition to having gained a new perspective because someone else pointed it out, it can be profound to realize that seeing a new perspective does not compromise one's original point of view at all. The duck does not cease to exist when the rabbit comes into view! Acknowledging a different way of thinking is crucial to the listening process. The practice of perspective-taking can be explored further by looking at Figure 3.2. Instead of asking the question "What is it?" ask, "What could it be?" There are no wrong answers, only different perspectives and maybe true curiosity.

Make Validation a Priority

Validation is an incredibly powerful and often underused strategy for respectful listening. It is closely related to true curiosity and perspective-taking because, in essence, it is about honoring another person. Listeners validate others when they use verbal and nonverbal language to show

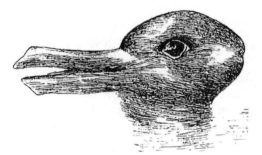

Figure 3-1 Rabbit/duck illusion.

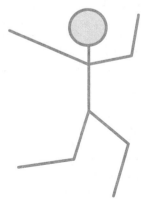

Figure 3-2 What do you see this figure doing?

they understand what the speaker is saying and why it is important to them. It has absolutely noth-ing to do with what the listener can or cannot, should or should not, will or will not do in response.

For example, consider a nurse working with a patient who has dementia and lives in a long-term care facility. The resident wants to go home or is "exit-seeking," a common experience, especially in the late afternoon and early evening when "sundowning" (increased confusion, frustration, and combativeness) tends to occur. Here is a conversation in which the nurse validates a male patient's feelings in such a circumstance:

Resident: I want to go home.

Nurse: You want to go home?

Resident: Yes, how do I get out of here?

Nurse: It sounds like you don't want to be here one bit!

Resident: I hate it here.

Nurse: I'm sorry it is so hard to be here.

At this point, the conversation could go in several different directions, and although there is no guarantee that continuing to validate the resident will eliminate his escalating frustration or even a physically threatening situation, it often does, and therefore it is better for everyone to try.

Consider how it might be a different experience for the resident if the nurse did not validate the patient, as with any of these responses:

Resident: I want to go home.

Nurse: You can't go home.

Resident: I want to go home.

Nurse: This is your home.

Resident: I want to go home.

Nurse: I'll get you some ice cream.

As shown in the first conversation, validation encourages the person to be part of the solu-tion rather than contribute to a power struggle. Validation demonstrates compassion and ac-knowledgement of another person's very existence. Nurses do not have to fix, change, or even believe the circumstances in order to validate another's experience. Offering ice cream, engaging in an activity, or walking with the resident to his room may all be very effective, too, but only *after* validation has occurred.

Validating is effective even when there are no verbal cues, such as when a patient who is unable to speak grimaces during the administration of antibiotic medication mixed in applesauce. This revealing facial expression offers the nurse a great opportunity to seek eye contact, provide a sim-ple light touch on an arm, and say, "I'm sorry. That tasted terrible didn't it? I'll get you some juice." Whether or not there is a conscious exchange of information, patients will feel honored and be more trusting. Remember, somewhere between 80% and 90% of communication is nonverbal.

Overall, validation will decrease power struggles and pave the way for calmer, more productive conversations.

Use Receptive Body Language, Tone, and Nonverbal Communication

All of the listening strategies can be enhanced by using receptive body language, tone, and non-verbal expressions. Because the vast majority of communication is nonverbal, facial expressions, physical stance, and tone of voice convey powerful messages from speakers and listeners. Lean-ing in toward or sitting next to someone suggests an interest in hearing what that person has to say, as opposed to towering over or standing in someone's personal space, which suggests a need to control or dominate the conversation. Nodding and offering occasional sounds such as "hmm" or "ahh" can indicate attentiveness and understanding that will contribute to the speaker's feelings of being heard.

In addition, listening includes paying attention to the body language, tone, and nonverbal communication of the person speaking. The patient who states, "I'm not in pain" while grimacing and the colleague who states, "I'd be happy to help" in an annoyed tone are providing mixed messages that warrant further probing. It is irresponsible for a nurse to document that a patient is denying pain and refusing pain medication without validating the patient's facial expression and seeking to understand more about what is going on with the patient. The patient may have a fear of addiction or of showing weakness, or may even worry about bothering the nurse, all which indicate the need for education and reassurance or perhaps a call to the physician to discuss alternative pain medicine. A much more professional and helpful manner of approaching the situation would be to say, "I hear you saying that you don't have any pain, and yet you seem as though you are in pain when you clutch your stomach and frown. Can you tell me more about what is going on?"

Remember that nonverbal communication may not always mean what it appears to mean. It may seem evident that a person standing with her arms crossed in front of her chest is showing resistance, when in fact the person is cold or trying to cover a drop of coffee spilled on her shirt earlier in the day. Clarifying why the person is crossing her arms is appropriate, whereas making an assumption is not: "I'm getting the sense you are angry by the way you're standing. Are you upset about something? Am I misunderstanding?"

Another way for a nurse to use nonverbal communication to show that she is paying attention is the intentional use of touch, which has been proved to be beneficial to patients (Conner & Howett, 2009). Placing a hand lightly on the arm of a patient who is anxiously awaiting surgery can be calming and reassuring. There may be times when hugging a patient or family member is perfectly appropriate and even therapeutic (e.g., a family member whose loved one has just passed away). Keep in mind that not everyone likes to be touched and that some may find it threatening, and there is always the possibility that someone could perceive a touch as having sexual implications. Watch for visual cues like facial grimaces or recoils from touch, and when in doubt, ask, "Is it okay if I touch your arm?"

Lastly, allowing for pauses or moments of silence in conversation gives feedback to the speaker that the listener is not in a rush. Silence also allows both parties the opportunity to think about what is being said.

Be Honest About Limitations

Infinite variables, including physiological, emotional, and intellectual stressors, may affect the listener. As important as listening is, there are times when one is not fully available, and there are places not conducive to a private conversation. It is much healthier to have ownership about limitations than to pretend to listen or shift priorities when more urgent duties are waiting. Finding the emotional energy and time to listen to a patient or colleague may or may not be realistic at any given moment, which should be conveyed honestly: "I'd really like to stop and listen to you right now, but I won't be able to concentrate because I'm not feeling well. I want to hear what you have to say. Can we schedule some time in the next couple of days?" The same idea can be applied to finding an appropriate place that feels safe to both parties.

The sender of information may also have extenuating circumstances, such as a clinical emergency or troubling personal matter, and may have difficulty transmitting information clearly and succinctly. Being mindful of what is or might be going on for others will model patience and is a great way to teach respectful listening.

Stay in the Present

Maintaining composure during stressful conversations is not easy. Mindfulness activities such as deep breathing or meditation help a person stay focused on the present, remain calm during a heated conversation, and recover more quickly from a tense exchange. Nurses with self-awareness will learn to notice when stress is increasing and can intentionally call on mindfulness practices to slow down an anxious reaction. One deep slow breath can help a person stay centered and in that moment. Developing a regular practice of relaxation such as meditation or yoga can help to decrease overall stress. If aware of increased stress but unable to calm down, one should take the opportunity to excuse oneself from the conversation and collect one's thoughts.

GRRRR: A MODEL FOR GREAT LISTENING

Becoming a better listener requires emotional intelligence (as presented in Chapter 2; see Goleman, 1995, 1998). At the same time, practicing listening skills will help to develop emotional intelligence competencies. Listening and emotional intelligence are intertwined with human behaviors and susceptible to personal limitations and organizational barriers. The model GRRRR for Great Listening is a formula designed to help the receiver in the mastery of listening. (Chapter 4 covers the SBAR model, which offers a framework that focuses on the sender of the message and the message itself.) GRRRR for Great Listening provides a structured guide for use when receiving important information about a patient, such as during a handoff (Boynton, 2009). The model makes the reporting of critical information a shared responsibility because it prompts the listener to contribute to a respectful climate for dialogue. Any efforts to encourage patients, consumers, and healthcare professionals to speak up will be more effective when they trust they will be listened to.

The acronym GRRRR is described as follows:

- Greeting: Set the tone for a professional dialogue with a kind hello and by using the other party's name: "Hi Beth, this is Mary, the nursing supervisor. How can I help?" This is a simple and respectful way to begin a conversation that may be stressful.

- Respectful listening: Let the other party finish sentences without interruption, but do make occasional acknowledgments, such as "okay" or "hmm." Allowing for brief pauses can ease anxiety and give the other party a chance to think and transmit critical information. If the communication takes place in person, make eye contact, nod, and use other receptive body language to promote rapport, even in the middle of an emergency.

- Reviewing: Summarize the information the speaker has conveyed to ensure that you understand the message correctly and to give the speaker a chance to correct or add any information. Inherent in validating, reviewing allows you to clarify your concerns and express additional thoughts without being intimidating or humiliating the other person. A few seconds spent doing so can help the speaker feel heard, respected, and ultimately understood.

- Recommending or Requesting (more information): Once the speaker is finished conveying his or her report and has been validated, and the message has been clarified, it is time to either make recommendations or request more information. Even if the recommendation differs from one suggested by the sender, it is important to maintain a collaborative approach and avoid put-downs: "A chest tube is a reasonable suggestion, and the objective information you've provided is great. However, this patient has some heart failure and that could be part of the problem. Let's do a chest x-ray and ABGs."

■ Rewarding: Rewarding the speaker for the information helps the person feel like a respected team player and is easily done with a simple acknowledgment: "Thanks for your call and attention to our patient's needs."

Confident Voices

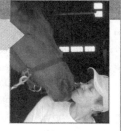

Pam Neff Montembeau, PT, DPT, CSCS
Physical Therapist

Listening

It seemed like an "ordinary" day in physical therapy school, filled with lectures, labs, and the occasional guest speaker. Little did I know that the guest speaker this day would influence my life so profoundly with his very first statement: "Your patients are your best teachers." Apologetically, I have forgotten his name now along with the specific topic on which he spoke that day. However, I do recall his white lab coat, slightly graying hair, and that humbly accurate statement. I somehow knew it was a "light bulb moment" for me. Since that day, and after more than 25 years as a practicing physical therapist, I am reminded almost daily how true that statement was and continues to be in my professional world, and how crucially important it is to any provider–patient relationship.

I believe it takes a village to heal a patient. Successful listening outcomes happen in healthcare when we listen with our eyes and ears, conduct face-to-face interactions, and respectfully touch and feel our patients to better appreciate the descriptive narrative they are telling us. An all-encompassing and collaborative healthcare team approach includes respectful provider–patient relationships, provider(provider relationships, and sometimes provider–family relationships. If the team members can truly understand the patient and the patient's reason for seeking healthcare, and can then unite all the pieces that make up medicine–providers, tests, medications, specialty care, care plan options, and so on), they get closer to optimal well-being outcomes for their patients.

One of the many gifts we receive from truly listening to our patients is what I call "privilege." What a privilege it is to embrace so many life stories and life lessons because we have crossed paths with someone we might not have otherwise met in our life. I am forever grateful to the speaker that day in physical therapy school, who in one statement spoke an immeasurable truth on the value of listening as a best practice in healthcare. I am a very lucky and privileged person.

Biography

Pam Neff Montembeau, PT, DPT, CSCS is a doctor of Physical Therapy in independent practice. She is the owner of Health Matters Physical Therapy, LLC, in Kittery, Maine.

RECEIVING FEEDBACK

One more area in which effective and respectful listening skills are crucial is in receiving feedback. Feedback is an ongoing part of the communication processes. Feedback—constructive or otherwise—may come out of a personnel evaluation, a conflict with a colleague, collaboration with a group, or a good friend's perspective. Listening effectively to feedback provides opportunities to build better relationships, resolve conflicts, and gain insight helpful for personal growth, but receiving feedback is not always easy. Here are some guidelines for how to listen to feedback and use it to the best advantage:

- Breathe. Especially when receiving harsh criticism, remember that you are a worthy person. Feedback is from the giver's perspective, and you can choose what to take in.
- Consider your choices. Is it a good or at least reasonable time and place for you to receive feedback? If not, inquire if there is a way to schedule a dialogue at a time that allows you to honor any needs you have regarding vulnerability, place, or other issues.
- Listen carefully and try to drop your defensiveness. Paraphrase the information you are receiving to make sure you understand the information. Validate what is being said and ask questions for clarity.
- Acknowledge the feedback. Let the speakers know you have heard them and that you will consider their feedback.
- Take time to sort out what you have heard. Give yourself time and space to assimilate and evaluate the information. Remember that it is not necessary to agree or disagree with the feedback. It is simply information. Let go of the need to justify, defend, or explain your actions. Do not over-internalize the feedback.
- Be honest with yourself. Use feedback as an opportunity to create greater awareness. Explore any feelings created by the feedback. Accept some discomfort in the process.
- Give yourself credit. Receiving feedback is hard work, and deciding to change or not change behavior based on feedback can be challenging. Give yourself credit for at least giving it proper consideration.

CASE STUDY

Matilda, a full-time RN working the 11:00 p.m. to 7:00 a.m. shift on the oncology unit of a large teaching hospital, arrives to work to find that concerns she had expressed about pain management for a new admission from the previous night have not been addressed. Matilda is worried that Mrs. Jones, who has stage IV lymphoma, is having preventable breakthrough pain. The 3:00 p.m. to 11:00 p.m. RN says he did not get a report from Linda, the day shift nurse, about pain, even though Matilda had noted her concerns in the patient's record as well as asked Linda personally to follow up. Matilda contacts the hospitalist immediately, and a new pain management protocol is instituted, but Matilda still feels the day shift nurse dropped the ball. As Matilda is leaving the next morning, she confronts Linda when she is getting off the elevator: "Why didn't you get on top of

Mrs. Jones's pain yesterday? She told me she suffered all day!" Linda is irritated and responds that Mrs. Jones was sleeping every time she went in and did not complain once about being in pain. She believes Matilda is overreacting. Matilda gives Linda a report for the rest of her patients and goes home still feeling angry.

Discussion Questions

1. List three situations in the case study in which respectful and effective listening could have prevented the outcome.
2. What kind of listening strategy is Linda using, and what suggestions would you give her in terms of developing more effective and respectful listening skills?
3. What might Matilda have done differently to promote more respectful and effective listening on Linda's part?
4. How do you think this conversation is likely to affect future conversations between Linda and Matilda?

SUMMARY

Listening is a skill that requires practice, emotional intelligence, and time. When done effectively and respectfully, listening enhances patient care, nurse job satisfaction, and workplace relationships. The essential skills and capacities for respectful listening are promoted by the Institute of Medicine (National Research Council, 2003) in its call for educators and licensing organizations to strengthen health professional training requirements in the delivery of patient-centered care. Health professionals are the conduits for responding to the unique needs, values, and preferences of individual patients and colleagues. Opportunities always exist for integrating understanding and compassion with clinical interventions and expertise. Effective and respectful listening is essential for patient-centered care and, further, is linked to improved outcomes such as better adherence to clinician recommendations and fewer diagnostic tests (Stewart et al., 2000).

Reflection Questions

1. In what ways are you an effective and respectful listener? Give an example of when these skills have resulted in a positive outcome for you, a patient, or your colleagues.
2. List one or two ways that you could further develop your ability to listen more effectively and respectfully.
3. Can you think of a time when you felt someone listened to you respectfully? What was that experience like?
4. Consider a time when you received constructive feedback from a nursing instructor, classmate, or other person involved in your nursing education. Measure your response against the tips for receiving feedback in this chapter. Describe how one or more of the tips might have helped improve the experience.

References

Beebe, S. A., Beebe, S. J., & Redmond, M. V. (2014). *Interpersonal communication: Relating to others* (7th ed.). Toronto, Ontario: Pearson Education Canada.

Boynton, B. (2009). How to improve your listening skills. *American Nurse Today, 4*(9), 50–51.

Conner, A., & Howett, M. (2009). A conceptual model of intentional comfort touch. *Journal of Holistic Nursing, 27*(2), 127–135.

Fisher, D. (1993). *Communication in organizations* (2nd ed.). St. Paul, MN: West Publishing.

Goleman, D. (1995). *Emotional intelligence: Why it can matter more than IQ*. New York: Bantam Books.

Goleman, D. (1998). *Working with emotional intelligence*. New York: Bantam Books.

National Research Council. (2003). *Health professions education: A bridge to quality*. Washington, DC: National Academies Press.

Stewart, M., Brown, J. B., Donner, A., McWhinney, I. R., Oates, J., Weston, W. W., & Jordan, J. (2000). The impact of patient-centered care on outcomes. *Journal of Family Practice, 49*(9), 796–804.

CHAPTER 4

Assertiveness

- Explain why assertiveness is a critical skill for nurse professionals
- Demonstrate use of the SBAR model to report a concern about a patient to a physician or nurse leader
- Explain the benefits and challenges of using I-statements
- Increase ability to give feedback effectively

- Assertiveness
- SBAR (situation, background, assessment, and recommendation) model
- I-statements
- Ownership

Nurses have valuable information and ideas that can positively affect patient care, policies, and protocols about care delivery and organizational processes. They also have their own needs, wants, and limitations. Nurses must be able to speak up confidently for patients and for themselves under stressful, highly charged emotional conditions and in environments where there are unequal power dynamics and resistance to or lack of skill in listening. Assertive communication (introduced in Chapter 1) is an important part of the behavioral approach to communication and supports safe care, positive workplaces, and rewarding careers.

This chapter identifies why assertiveness is important in nurse practice settings and helps students to develop their capacity to show ownership. In addition, SBAR, a common model of structured communication, is examined, and the uses and challenges of I-statements in developing and practicing assertiveness are discussed. Finally, students will learn guidelines for giving constructive feedback as an important communication tool useful in forming collaborative relationships, managing conflict, and developing leadership skills.

WHY ASSERTIVENESS IS VITAL

Assertiveness is often associated with an individual's ability to speak up confidently, which can be challenging for many nurses. Assertiveness often requires taking risks and being accountable, and it requires personal growth in emotional intelligence such as developing self-awareness, self-confidence, and motivation. For many nurses, the road to assertiveness also involves challenging core beliefs that have been shaped by life experiences, family, and ethnicity and culture. It can take years of practice. Success may ebb and flow depending on work and personal stressors that may influence one's confidence level. Learning to be assertive will also be hindered or helped by the quality of listening as well as the degree of trust and respect that prevail in the organizational culture in which a nurse practices. In their discussion on creating a "code of mutual respect," Suzanne Gordon, Patrick Mendenhall, and Bonnie Blair O'Connor (2013) advise that, "Since teamwork means that all members of the team, no matter where they are positioned, must feel free to speak up, psychological safety—the sense that people will not be blown off, humiliated, belittled, made fun of, or simply ignored when they raise critical issues or express their perspectives—is key" (pp. 62–63).

Some nurses are more assertive by nature, whereas others will find the skills more challenging to develop. Nevertheless, nurses who have passive, passive-aggressive, or aggressive tendencies must work at becoming assertive communicators in order to develop and maintain a high standard of professionalism.

Nurses at all levels have endless opportunities to practice, develop, and role-model assertiveness. There are several areas in which assertiveness is vital:

- Speaking up for patients
- Building and maintaining relationships with colleagues
- Speaking up for oneself

Speaking Up for Patients

Communication failures are consistently linked to root causes of medical errors (The Joint Commission, 2014). Therefore, speaking up for patients and acting as an advocate are the most obvious need for practicing assertiveness in nursing. Doing so requires knowledge, confidence, and a willingness to step up and report concerns to colleagues and physicians, despite fears of being wrong, inconveniencing others, or even being disrespected. Ensuring that the physician is aware of a patient's allergy, stopping a procedure because of a potential error, and reminding a colleague to wash hands before a dressing change are all examples of using assertiveness to advocate for patients.

The act of a nurse speaking up for a patient can in turn encourage a patient to be assertive. The following scenarios demonstrate examples of nurses speaking up and their patients finding their own assertiveness because of it, leading to successful patient outcomes. In the first scenario, a patient comes to an outpatient clinic with a recurrent sinus infection. The doctor hands the nurse a prescription for Bactrim with one refill. The nurse thinks for a moment about a brief phone conversation she had with the patient the previous day. As the doctor heads off, the nurse calls out, "Wait! That patient is allergic to sulfa. What alternative antibiotic would you like to prescribe?" When the patient overhears the nurse's question, she confirms it and shares her experience with joint pain while on the drug. With that knowledge, the doctor prescribes a different antibiotic. In the second scenario, a patient confides in a nurse that he is having second thoughts about a third round of chemotherapy and is interested in learning more about hospice care. The nurse could be assertive by reporting the patient's concerns to the physician or by encouraging the patient to express his concerns to the doctor. She decides to do both: "It is important for Dr. Jones to know about your concerns. I'll let him know you are having second thoughts, and suggest he stop by so you two can talk more about it. Does that should okay?" In both cases, the nurse is assertive in making sure the physician gets the information, and the patient is encouraged to do the same. While patients can certainly benefit from being assertive, it is not a requirement that they do so. However, as healthcare systems become more transparent, the role of patients and families as collaborative partners is shifting, making assertiveness by patients more necessary (this will be discussed more completely in Chapter 6).

Confident Voices

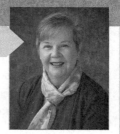

Patricia Iyer , MSN, RN, LRCC
President of the Pat Iyer Group

Don't Let Them Down

You are a student nurse assigned to the labor and delivery unit. You've been taught to interpret the electronic fetal monitoring strip. You notice a sudden drop in heart rate to the 60s. You know this needs to be reported. When you enter the nursing station, you see the patient's obstetrician. He is sitting in the nursing station with the head nurse on his lap, and they are laughing in an intimate way. They look at you, and he asks in an annoyed manner, "What do *you* want?" You hesitate but then clearly request the head nurse to recheck the fetal heart rate. She also obtains a heart rate in the 60s. The team goes into action, concludes the umbilical cord is being compressed, performs an emergency cesarean section, and delivers a healthy infant. This is not a hypothetical story—it happened to me when I was in nursing school.

For the last 26 years, I have developed a deep understanding of the factors that lead to medical errors. My legal nurse consulting experience has exposed me to many legal cases that would never have happened if only one person had spoken up on behalf of the patient. Astute observations, clear communication, and professional teamwork save lives and improve patient outcomes, decrease the risk for preventable adverse events affecting patients, and increase job satisfaction. Nurses are more likely to stay in their positions when they feel like a valued member of the team.

What stands in the way of this type of teamwork?

- **The power structure in the workplace.** Physicians have traditionally been seen as the key players responsible for bringing revenue (patients) to the hospital. Some specialties (e.g., cardiac surgery, neurosurgery) create particularly lucrative revenue opportunities.
- **Leadership.** It takes a strong leader to stand up to a powerful physician who crosses the line by behaving in a demeaning way to others. A cardiac surgeon stormed into an operating room in his street clothes and berated a surgeon who was in the middle of cardiac surgery. The hospital chose not to renew his contract because of his inability to control his temper. This was an act of courage that gained the administration the respect of the staff.
- **Ineffective conflict resolution.** Many healthcare providers have not been taught how to manage conflict, stand up for themselves, or assertively communicate with other providers.

So what can you do? Suppose you are treated in a harsh, demeaning way by another member of the healthcare team. Often we are caught off guard when this

Continued

Confident Voices—cont'd

happens, and in hindsight wish we had responded differently. Think through what happened and how you felt about it. Sometimes all it takes is seeking out the person involved in the interaction and discussing how you felt about what happened. Speak to your nurse manager, preceptor, or more experienced staff members to gain some insight on the situation and how you might handle it differently. By no means should you silently take abuse.

You should be able to expect to work in a healthcare environment that respects the contributions of all professionals, where you can practice in an environment of respect. You are responsible for speaking up—for yourself and for your patients. Your patients rely on you to give them attention and get them attention. They require rapid resolution of conflicts. They count on you. Don't let them down.

Biography

Patricia Iyer, MSN, RN, LNCC, has spent 26 years evaluating medical malpractice and personal injury cases as a legal nurse consultant. A prolific author, she has written, coauthored, or coedited more than 185 books, articles, chapters, case studies, and online courses. She is particularly interested in helping nurses act as patient advocates by speaking on behalf of their patients. Her website is www.PatIyer.com.

Building and Maintaining Relationships With Colleagues

Practicing assertiveness and avoiding passive, passive-aggressive, and aggressive behavior helps in building and maintaining collaborative relationships among colleagues. The nurse who clearly states she has an idea that might help a colleague's patient is demonstrating assertiveness by offering a useful insight to her colleagues about another's patient's care: "I had a very difficult time getting a good vein for Mrs. Moore's IV on admission, and she was very anxious. If she needs a new one, and you're still unsure of your technique, it might make sense to get the IV team up here."

Assertiveness among colleagues can also improve a working environment, as shown in the following scenario: As the second shift is beginning on the medical-surgical unit, two nurses are talking about a newer nurse who has yet to arrive. One of the nurses comments that she does not think this nurse is going to make it on this unit: "She asks the same questions over and over again, and never gets out on time. She's spending way too much time with patients, and last week it took her 2 hours to admit someone!" The nurse she's talking to has similar feelings, but he decides to act on them in a more positive way: "I understand where you are coming from and wonder if we could help her by offering some constructive feedback. It could help her to become more confident and get things done a little faster. She seems pretty sharp and very compassionate to me." This nurse manages to be diplomatic in validating the other nurse's concerns yet does not take sides against the new nurse. His assertive approach is an important step toward creating a more respectful environment, and other nurses could learn a lot about assertiveness from him.

Assertiveness is the best way to stop passive-aggressive gossiping. It would be nice to think that this nurse would have spoken up no matter what, but certain power dynamics can compromise such efforts. What if the problem nurse is actually the unit manager? A nurse may worry about facing repercussion in that instance. To practice assertiveness, nurses need to understand what leadership support exists—or does not.

Speaking Up for Oneself

Lastly, showing assertiveness by speaking up for oneself is an important component of staying healthy and providing safe care. Nursing is a profession of service and compassion, both of which are honorable commitments. However, this does not mean that the needs of nurses should be ignored or undervalued, especially chronically. Historically, the culture of nursing has included an element of martyrdom, which is not healthy.

The following scenario demonstrates how nurses can use assertiveness to improve self-care (which will be discussed in more detail later in this chapter and in Chapter 8): A nurse is 2 hours away from the end of four back-to-back 12-hour day shifts in an acute care rehabilitation hospital. She did not stop for lunch, although she grabbed half a sandwich from a colleague. She has a complicated discharge to complete, including at least 1 hour's worth of patient teaching and paperwork as well as several more medications to administer. She is also scheduled to work the next day from 7:00 a.m. to 7:00 p.m. The nurse manager approaches and asks her to take on the admission of new patient on his way in. The nurse takes a deep breath and says, "I'm sorry, but I'm maxed out. I haven't had lunch and will be lucky if I get out on time as it is. Please try to get someone else to help."

There are endless variations to this scenario in day-to-day practice. Some individuals will never be able to stay late because of child care issues. Some units always have enough staff to cover sick calls, so their nurses are rarely asked to stay late. Whatever the situation, nurses need to decide at what point and in what circumstances they honor the needs of the unit before their own. In addition, nurses must respect limits that others set even when they are different from their own. Setting limits like this is hard but necessary for every nurse and, in the long run, benefits colleagues, patients, family, and even the organization. A nurse's ability to provide safe care is compromised by consecutive shifts and fatigue. By being assertive and setting limits, nurses will be happier, healthier, and more rested.

Consultant Commentary

If we are going to be successful in teaching nurses to be assertive in all ways, we need to recognize how hard it can be to learn and the importance of psychological safety. I consider myself to be quite assertive at this point in my career, but that does not mean it has been easy or comes easily now. A few years ago, I was giving my very first keynote address, at the Washington State Nurses Association National Conference. There were about 100 nurse leaders in the audience. Standing there with my microphone, PowerPoint presentation, and some anxiety, I started by sharing a story about asserting myself over staffing and a safety concern just 2 weeks earlier in my per diem role as a staff RN. As I told the attendees, I had found out in the middle of a shift that I was supposed to be supervising a medication technician, who was giving medications on an adjacent unit. A patient had a skin tear, and the technician came to me because she was told I was the nurse supervising her and she needed me to take care of the patient, fill out the incident report, and call the family and

Continued

Consultant Commentary—cont'd

physician. I was surprised that I was supposed to be supervising the technician because I already had my hands full with my own patients. I contacted the nursing supervisor, who was also very busy, and we completed the extra work together. But I went home an hour late and also angry.

That night, I thought a lot about how I should address my concerns. The next day, I went in a few minutes early and shared my thoughts with the scheduler. I explained that I did not feel it was safe and I did not have the time to be supervising another staff member on a different unit. The scheduler told me that he "couldn't make any promises." So I took a deep breath and went to the director of nurses. My mouth was dry, and I could feel my heart racing when I told her my concerns. Fortunately, she found my concerns valid, and I was never put in that situation again.

Even though I teach assertiveness and speak in front of groups of people, it was a very hard thing to do. I share that story hoping that it will encourage students to be easy on themselves and each other as they develop assertiveness.

SBAR MODEL

The idea that nurses should be assertive has always been a part of nursing education. After all, reporting concerns about a patient's clinical status to a nurse supervisor or physician is an integral part of the job. But the complexity of it and its importance in patient safety gained more attention in the latter part of the 20th century as awareness grew about the implications of communication in medical errors. In 2005, The Joint Commission recommended that healthcare facilities include assertiveness training for nurses (The Joint Commission, 2005). One of the strategies that healthcare leaders developed in response and that is used by many facilities today is the **SBAR (situation, background, assessment, and recommendation) model** for transmitting critical information.

Standard communication models are especially helpful in creating common patterns for sharing information, as tools for learning and practicing skills, and to fall back on when facing stressful situations. SBAR is the most prominent model that has emerged in healthcare over the past 10 years as a result of addressing patient safety issues that stem from miscommunication.

SBAR originated in the military and is being used more and more in healthcare to standardize and clarify reporting efforts in which critical information is being transmitted. It is the communication process of choice at many facilities and helps to standardize a way of reporting concerns and observations about patients to physicians or supervisors. It is designed to frame all necessary information succinctly and in a logical order along with a suggestion as to what the next step should be.

SBAR helps convey critical information by requiring the clinician to pull together relevant information so that the physician or other provider can make a decision. In doing so, it promotes a critical thinking process that helps a nurse or other healthcare professional prepare to contact a physician or higher-level practitioner with clear and succinct information. In terms of addressing underlying communication problems, its focus is on the sender of information and the message itself.

Here is an example of a nurse using the SBAR model to contact a physician about a patient:

Situation: Hello, Dr. Jones. This is Nurse Smith calling from the Med-Surg Unit at ABC Hospital regarding Mrs. Brown. I'm calling because I'm concerned that the area of cellulitis on her right calf is spreading.

Background: She is 74 years old and has a history of type 2 diabetes, which according to the ED notes has been under control with oral medications. She was admitted last night from the ED for cellulitis of her left calf and started on IV penicillin.

Assessment: The area of redness and swelling last night was circled and documented as 12 cm ($\times$ 20 cm and is spreading in all directions. I measured 15 $\times$ 25 cm, her temperature is 101° F, and her blood glucose is 268. Her vital signs are stable. She had one dose of IV PCN 500 mg in the ED and has had two more since being admitted to the floor. Her calf is swollen, red, and tender to light touch. She does not seem to be responding to the antibiotic therapy, and her condition is worsening.

Recommendation: I think she may need a different antibiotic and maybe blood cultures, and/or a sliding scale insulin regimen.

Recent pioneers and researchers Michael Leonard, Audrey Lyndon, Jill Morgan, and Ansley Stone discussed the increased use of SBAR in an Institute for Healthcare Improvement (IHI; 2014b) broadcast, including how it is helping nurses to raise clinical concerns to the next level of authority. They also discuss growing awareness of weaknesses, namely that SBAR lacks a focus on listening and that nurses still struggle with the recommendation part of the model.

As the SBAR model gains traction in the industry, variations are emerging, including SBARR (McMillan, 2010), in which the second "R" stands for "read back," intended to remind nurses to review and confirm orders; and ISBAR, in which the "I" stands for "identifying," intended to remind nurses to properly identify everyone involved in a handoff (IHI, 2014a). There are other communication models emerging with various degrees of use, and the Agency for Healthcare Research and Quality (2013) provides a comprehensive list as well.

Ultimately, the success of any communication model will depend to a great extent on the individual's ability to speak up and listen as well as on the workplace culture.

I-STATEMENTS

One of the most effective ways to develop assertiveness is with the use of **I-statements**. An I-statement is a communication method that encourages speakers to show **ownership** about a concern, want, or need. It includes identification of emotions and invites other speakers to participate in the conversation in a collaborative fashion. It helps steer people away from blaming others because it requires individuals to recognize their part in a conflict or difficult situation. All these factors make I-statements a valuable tool in building assertiveness.

Many nurses have some knowledge about I-statements but may not use them frequently in the workplace. It is not unusual for nurses to get caught up in blaming others or becoming defensive rather than asserting themselves and owning their part in a conflict. Consider a scenario in which a highly educated and experienced nurse is frustrated with the lack of orientation new nurses are getting in the intensive care unit in which she works. She seems to be in a power struggle with her manager, who has advised her that the decision has been made and there is no budget for additional training. Over and over, she keeps saying, "They need more training," without it getting her anywhere. This nurse is worried that patients are at risk and feels liable for the new nurses' actions. If she had initiated a conversation with her manager that began with her concerns (e.g., "I think the patients are at risk and that I might be liable") rather than being adamant about the solution, she may have had a more productive conversation. Instead, she came off as angry and could not get to a place where she could show ownership and invite collaborative problem-solving.

Ownership and assertiveness go hand in hand and inherently involve self-esteem, self-awareness, and self-respect. However, rather than framing a problem from their perspective, many nurses find it easier or safer to point out what someone else is doing. By doing so, they:

- Avoid responsibility for their own feelings
- Blame and/or judge others
- Present opinions as if they are facts
- Do not allow room for other perspectives
- Are authoritarian or controlling
- Tend to delay conflict resolution
- Can be manipulative
- Offer sweeping generalizations

For example, consider the following statements:

"You make me so angry when you leave a pile of charts out on the counter."

and

"I'm upset by this pile of charts on the counter. I have no space to work, can't find charts I need, and I worry about confidentiality. I'd appreciate it if you would be more careful about this."

The first statement is likely to escalate the situation by blaming and being argumentative. The second statement is much more respectful, builds the relationship, and shows ownership— an ideal example of an effective I-statement.

When used properly, I-statements have many advantages. They:

- Increase the chance of effective communication and collaboration
- Lead to more efficient problem-solving and conflict resolution
- Validate many different perspectives
- Build and nourish relationships
- Build self-awareness, self-respect, and self-efficacy

Using I-statements can be awkward and cumbersome at first, but with practice they can give the speaker a genuine sense of ownership of their thoughts and are particularly helpful in stressful situations. To develop skill in using I-statements, it helps to use the following sentence formats when speaking:

I feel _____

When you _____

Because _____

I would like _____

To help in deciding whether using an I-statement in a particular situation would be helpful, use the following self-reflective checklist. The more checks that apply to the situation, the more useful an I-statement will be:

- I'm trying to repair or build this relationship.
- I want a solution that will work for all involved.
- I value and respect my own opinion.
- I value and respect the opinions of others involved.
- I am willing to disclose an appropriate amount of personal information.
- I am open to ideas from others involved.
- I am willing to compromise or collaborate.

Making Effective I-statements

The effectiveness of I-statements depends on the relationship between the people having the conversation. If there is a basis of mutual trust and respect in place, an I-statement will naturally lead to collaboration. If there is tension, I-statements may help to diminish resentment and defensiveness making effective collaboration more likely.

Let's look at a scenario in which an I-statement is effective: A supervisor has been giving a nurse more and more work over a period of several weeks and is now delegating her yet another project. Using an I-statement, the nurse approaches another colleague: "I'm overwhelmed with this new project because I'm overloaded with my current assignments. Can you help share the work?" With this statement, the nurse shows ownership and suggests a way to solve the problem. The nurse could have responded more negatively, saying to her colleague: "My supervisor is driving me crazy. She keeps piling on more and more work and doesn't care how it affects me. I can't stand working for her." In that case, there would be no ownership of the problem and instead an attempt to build an alignment with a third person against the leader.

Let's now consider how the conflict might be addressed from the leader's perspective using an I-statement: "I'm concerned that this patient assignment is creating a lot of stress for you. I can see that you are working really hard. How can I help?" This approach builds a positive relationship and encourages collaborative problem-solving. Asking the staff member what the supervisor can do to help shows assertiveness and promotes a climate in which asking for help is expected. The supervisor would have set a much different tone if she instead said something like the following: "If you need help, you are going to have to ask for it. I don't have the time or energy to coddle you. No one offered me any help when I worked on this floor." In this case, the leader may be holding onto old resentment and seeking validation for her bad experiences. Although there may be compassion for her experience, this approach is not respectful and contributes to a vicious cycle of passive-aggressive communication and behavior.

The Challenges of I-Statements

As the previous examples show, using I-statements can be very helpful when needing to communicate assertively or when under pressure. However, the format can be awkward and interfere with the natural flow of dialogue. This challenge should be temporary because the intended point of practicing I-statements is to develop a sense of ownership and respect for others. As nurses master this, the actual language matters less, and sincerity and assertiveness will come across in tone, body language, content, and actions.

Another challenge in using I-statements is that ownership of a problem may involve some risk taking in terms of revealing private information to others. How much each individual decides to share has personal and professional ramifications. A nurse's varying relationships with patients, colleagues, and leaders call for different approaches to being open and vulnerable. For example, "I'm upset about your tone for personal reasons" is quite different from "I'm a nervous wreck because your tone reminds me of my ex-husband and all of the abusive relationships I've been in."

One of the trickiest areas in which to practice I-statements is within provider–patient relationships, for these primary reasons:

1. Patients are in a dependent position. A nurse's role requires that he or she provide care and expertise for health and comfort of patients who are vulnerable.

2. Nurses must be aware of what their feelings are and where they are coming from. This includes awareness of any secondary gains they may get from patients being dependent on them. Feeling a sense of accomplishment because of a successful intervention or feedback from a patient is fine, but standards of care rather than feeling good should drive the intervention. Further, what the nurse thinks is helpful and what a patient thinks is helpful may be very different.

3. Nurses must be able to discern what is appropriate to share with patients and what is not. This does not mean nurses should bury feelings but rather that they should find alternate resources for support.

Nurses should also be careful about telling patients what they need, as, for example, in this statement: "You need to be honest with me about your chest pain. I take every complaint of pain very seriously." Admittedly, the historical standard is that healthcare professionals preside over patients rather than collaborate with them. However, telling others what they need promotes dependency rather than empowerment. Patients may always have some needs that can be met by nurses and other healthcare professionals, but it will be a healthier dependence if they, to the best of their abilities, are the ones who identify those needs and ask for help. Helping patients to identify their needs may increase engagement and improve outcomes. A better way to convey concern and empower this patient might sound like this: "I need you to be honest with me about your chest pain. I take every complaint seriously and want to make sure you are getting the best treatment. Your description of symptoms is really important."

. Nurses also have to be careful about blaming patients for their feelings, as can be sensed in this nurse's comment: "You don't follow instructions and keep coming back with problems that could have been prevented if you were listening." A more appropriate way for the nurse to show her frustration in this scenario might be for her to say: "When you come back to the clinic with problems that could have been prevented, I feel like I'm not doing a very good job of teaching you how to take care of your diabetes. Do you have some thoughts on how we could work together more effectively?" The use of I-statements with patients can be an effective and nonthreatening way to set limits and improve compliance. What nurses share about themselves or ask patients to do for them requires prudence. When in doubt, run it by a colleague or privately reflect, "Is it fair to ask this patient to do this for me, or is it more appropriate for me to express my concerns to a team member or supervisor?"

The final thing to be aware of in forming I-statements is not to use them to disguise "You-statements." Consider these comments:

"I feel like you have never respected me and never will."

"I feel like you are a snobby know-it-all."

Both start out with "I feel . . .," but neither shows ownership or respect. It is easy to fall into this trap if a nurse is still learning the I-statement model or if the speaker is especially hurt, angry, or vulnerable. Disguised comments such as these can be confusing, abusive, and give the practice of I-statements a bad name.

Confident Voices

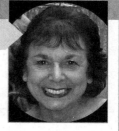

Terri Goodman, PhD, RN, CNOR
Owner of Terri Goodman & Associates

Welcome to the Internship

Communication plays a definitive role in the process of developing the knowledge base and skills to work in the perioperative arena with competence and confidence. For most nursing graduates, the operating room is a whole new world, not an extension of their nursing school experience. It is hard for them to imagine that they will master enough of the knowledge base, clinical practice, and technology to function independently in 6 months. My job as the facilitator of their success is to empower *them* to make that happen. The key to their success is *speaking up* and *speaking out*.

On the first day, I face a group of bright young nurses thoroughly convinced that 6 months is much too short a time for them to become competent perioperative nurses. They stare at me with apprehension and wait for me to start teaching. I smile back into those wide eyes and say, "Welcome to the internship. First let me tell you that you are not students, and this is not school. You are licensed perioperative nurses; you are my colleagues, and it is my job to facilitate your success. It is your job to let me know what you need. You control the outcome of this learning experience by making sure that I provide the best learning environment for you and the opportunities that you need to achieve competence." That is quite a new perspective for most new graduates—the idea of being in charge, of being empowered to speak up and ask for what you need, takes a bit of getting used to.

I start each class by asking, "What help do you need to understand the material?" or "What skills need the most practice today?" The interns learn quickly that by speaking up they can tailor classes to their needs. Following a day in the clinical environment, I ask, "How did it go in the OR yesterday?" That never fails to elicit both positive stories—a wonderful experience with a surgeon who loves to teach or a preceptor who let them do everything they could—and negative stories—a disappointing day in a room where they were ignored or berated or missed out on opportunities to learn. Re-scripting the disappointing scenarios helps the interns realize their responsibility for facilitating the desired outcome by communicating their needs. Role-playing effective communication builds confidence and trust that communicating works. The interns learn to tell new preceptors what skills they have mastered

Continued

and to ask for specific learning opportunities. They also learn to thank everyone who has participated in their learning.

Respectful communication earns the interns some level of respect among their new colleagues. With the confidence that comes from taking charge of their learning environment, they find it less difficult to speak out, ask questions, and share best practices that promote patient safety. They are less hesitant to report a break in sterile technique or to insist that the alcohol prep be allowed to dry before draping the patient. One intern was confident enough to point out to a surgeon that the x-rays were mounted backward and that it was the left shoulder, not the right, that should be draped for the procedure. These interns have identified that developing respectful, collegial relationships is based on good communication, and that communication is key to getting what they want and need, solving problems, and promoting patient safety.

Biography

Terri Goodman, PhD, RN, CNOR, owns Terri Goodman & Associates, an approved provider of continuing nursing education, and is program facilitator for the Hospital Corporation of America, North Texas perioperative internship program. She is a perioperative nurse and holds leadership positions in organizations at the local, state, and national levels. Dr. Goodman is actively involved in efforts to achieve the Institute of Medicine recommendations for the future of nursing. She speaks nationally and publishes frequently.

PROVIDING FEEDBACK

One final but important way to develop assertiveness skills is through giving feedback. As noted in Chapter 3, feedback is an ongoing part of the communication process, and not only is feedback often hard to hear, it also can be difficult to give. Worries about rejection, retaliation, and hurting another's feelings contribute to avoiding or having trepidation about offering feedback. Yet ultimately, feedback demonstrates a respect for others, is important for learning how behaviors are perceived by others, and provides opportunities for personal and professional growth. There is an art to giving constructive feedback, and assertiveness is an inherent part of it. The following guidelines help to make the process respectful and meaningful:

- **Be kind and helpful.** Check in with your own intentions about offering feedback. Helping someone grow and learn is much different from putting someone in his or her place. Accept that there will be some discomfort in the process.
- **Check to see if feedback is wanted.** If you are not offering feedback that concerns a patient's safety or are in a leadership position in which giving feedback is part of your job,

ask if the feedback is wanted. If there is room for choice around time and place, it can be helpful to honor that as well. Consider approaching the person first and saying: "I have some feedback for you. Are you open hearing it?" If the answer is no, respect the person's decision.

- **Look for opportunities to include ownership.** Keep in mind that your feedback is based on your observation and to some extent what it means to you. For example, rather than saying, "You're so negative and angry," it shows more ownership to say, "My sense is that you are angry and it feels like negative energy to me."

- **Be specific and do not judge or exaggerate.** Give feedback without using words that indicate judgment. Do not use labels or exaggerate. Avoid loaded expressions such as "never" and "always."

- **Focus on concern for the person and behaviors that can be changed.** Monitor any attachment to being right and focus on the ways in which the person might be able to change.

- **Check the listener's perception.** Ask a follow-up question to see if the message has been accurately heard because the message sent is not always the message received. The feedback may need to be presented differently.

- **Ask questions.** In addition to sharing your thoughts, ask the person his or her opinions. Allow the receiver to suggest changes in behavior before you offer options.

CASE STUDY

Regina and David are certified nursing assistants (CNAs) working in a long-term care facility. One night on shift together, Regina calls out for help while transferring a patient from her wheelchair to bed. No one responds, and she transfers the patient by herself. Afterward, she storms out of the room and says angrily to the charge nurse, "I asked David for help, and he ignored me." David overhears the complaint and, with his hands on his hips, exclaims, "That's a lie! You did not signal for help. A call light goes on, and Regina walks away to answer it. "She's lying," David repeats to the charge nurse. "Can I go on my dinner break?" While on break, David tells colleagues that Regina is awful to work with and makes up lies about other people; he warns them to watch their backs. Shortly later, when Regina is on break, she tells other colleagues how lazy David is.

Discussion Questions

1. How would you assess Regina's assertiveness? What would have been a more assertive way for her to express her concerns?
2. How would you describe David's response? How could he reframe his response with some ownership?
3. How might this tension affect the care patients are receiving?
4. How might Regina and David's conflict affect the charge nurse's time?
5. What other ramifications might occur from this lack of respectful communication?

SUMMARY

Assertiveness is an important yet complicated aspect of communication and can have ramifications on safety, compliance, teamwork, and job satisfaction. Being assertive is essential to individual and professional growth. It may become easier with practice but can be hard to learn. Areas in which nurses must be assertive include speaking up for patients and oneself, building productive relationships, and giving constructive feedback, all of which are necessary for healthy workplaces and safe care. I-statements are an effective tool for developing assertiveness and contribute greatly to collaborative cultures. The more nurses can integrate ownership into their language, the more likely they will have their own needs met and the more respectful communication will be.

Reflection Questions

1. How would you rate your ability to be assertive in advocating for your patients? How would you rate your ability to be assertive in advocating for yourself? If there is any difference, what might be the explanation?

2. Have you ever had an I-statement backfire? Is there anything you would do differently given insights from this chapter?

3. Can you think of a conflict you have with a work colleague in which you could try out I-statements? How could you prepare for initiating the conversation?

4. Can you think of an opportunity in which you could practice giving constructive feedback to a classmate? How might this affect your ongoing education together?

References

Agency for Healthcare Research and Quality. (2013). TeamSTEPPS: Team strategies and tools to enhance performance and patient safety. Retrieved from www.ahrq.gov/professionals/education/curriculum-tools/teamstepps/instructor/essentials/pocketguide.html

Gordon, S., Mendenhall, P., & O'Connor, B. B. (2013). Beyond the checklist: What else health care can learn from aviation teamwork and safety. Ithaca, NY: Cornell University Press.

The Joint Commission. (2005). The Joint Commission guide to improving staff communication. Oakbrook Terrace, IL: The Joint Commission.

The Joint Commission. (2014). Sentinel event. Retrieved from www.jointcommission.org/sentinel_event.aspx

Institute for Healthcare Improvement. (2014a). ISBAR tip trick. Retrieved from www.ihi.org/resources/Pages/Tools/ISBARTripTick.aspx

Institute for Healthcare Improvement. (2014b). WIHI: SBAR: Structured communication and psychological safety in health care [audio and video]. Retrieved from www.ihi.org/resources/Pages/AudioandVideo/WIHISBARStructuredCommunicationandPsychologicalSafetyinHealthCare.aspx

McMillan, L. R. (2010). Utilizing SBARR: Using peer reviewers in a low-fidelity lab exercise. Retrieved from qsen.org/utilizing-sbarr-using-peer-reviewers-in-a-low-fidelity-lab-exercise

Why Successful Nurse Communication Is Critical

Part II reinforces why a behavioral approach to communication is essential in healthcare, particularly for addressing critical issues such as safe care, optimal patient experience, respectful workplace cultures, and long-term and rewarding careers. First, students will explore the statistics that make up and the causes behind the alarming persistence of medical and nursing errors. Next, they will delve into the nature of therapeutic relationships and patient experience and determine how to deal with workplace abuse. Finally, they will be given the incentive and tools for incorporating self-care into their commitment to nursing practice.

CHAPTER 5

Patient Safety

LEARNING OUTCOMES

- Discuss how key reports by the Institute of Medicine and various journals have highlighted serious problems in patient safety
- Identify organizations investigating issues with patient safety
- Explain how root cause analysis of sentinel events provides evidence supporting the need for nursing education to include development of effective and respectful communication skills
- Identify communication skills associated with categories and subcategories of root causes of sentinel events
- Explain how assertiveness and respectful listening will contribute to safe nursing care

KEY TERMS

- Patient safety
- Quality of care
- Sentinel event
- Adverse event
- Root cause analysis

Safe care should be an inherent part of every nursing intervention, treatment, and recommendation. Yet, although students of all healthcare professions are taught how to safely provide care using their respective expertise, in the real world, the incidence of errors is astronomically high. Solutions to date have made only a marginal impact and fall woefully short of the goal of making healthcare as safe as possible. Truly fixing the problem means changing the underlying human dynamics behind individual and organizational behavior, which are often difficult to measure, predict, and change. As students will learn in this chapter, the evidence exists to support a behavioral approach to communication as part of the solution to persistent problems with patient safety.

Students will examine patient safety through a lens that highlights the importance of communication and behavior in providing safe, quality care. This chapter begins by examining a brief history of patient safety and identifying major organizations associated with patient safety, statistics involving medical and nursing errors, and root causes and root cause analysis of sentinel events. Students will then be shown underlying causes of sentinel events and their correlation with communication and human behavior. Without this knowledge, the critical links between mistakes and communication may remain hidden from view, and long-term effective solutions may remain elusive.

DEFINING PATIENT SAFETY

In order for nurses to understand the role of communication and behavior in **patient safety**, they must have complete comprehension of the concept. A simple yet powerful definition of the term *patient safety* comes from the Institute of Medicine (IOM): "The prevention of harm caused by errors of commission and omission" (Aspden, Corrigan, Wolcott, & Erickson, 2004, p. 333). This definition highlights and promotes the commitment of all nurses to provide safe care.

A second, more complicated definition by the Agency for Healthcare Research and Quality (AHRQ) deems patient safety as "a discipline in the healthcare professions that applies safety science methods toward the goal of achieving a trustworthy system of healthcare delivery. We also define patient safety as an attribute of healthcare systems that minimizes the incidence and impact of adverse events and maximizes recovery from such events" (Emanuel et al., 2008, p. 19). This definition focuses on science but also on trustworthiness, the latter requiring ownership, positive workplace relationships, and collaboration.

A third definition, which invites consideration of individual and organizational behavior, comes from the Quality and Safety Education for Nurses (QSEN) Institute: "Minimize(ing) risk of harm to patients and providers through both system effectiveness and individual performance" (Cronenwett et al., 2007, p. 128).

To paint a complete picture of patient safety, **quality of care** must be included. The IOM considers patient safety "indistinguishable from the delivery of quality healthcare" (Aspden et al., 2004, p. 5) and describes quality of care as "the degree to which health services for individuals and populations increase the likelihood of desired health outcomes and are consistent with current professional knowledge" (IOM, 2001, p. 232). Nurses cannot provide quality care if the care they are providing is not safe.

A BRIEF HISTORY OF PATIENT SAFETY

The phrase "do no harm" is associated with the Hippocratic Oath (Edelstein, 1943), written thousands of years ago, and was echoed by Florence Nightingale in the mid-1800s (Nightingale, 1859). It was not until the turn of the 21st century, however, that an awareness of the magnitude of harm being caused in medicine and nursing began to take shape among healthcare professionals and in the public eye.

In 1999, the IOM published the groundbreaking report, *To Err Is Human: Building a Safer Health System* (Kohn, Corrigan, & Donaldson, 2000). This report, shocking at the time, estimated that 44,000 to 98,000 people die annually as a result of medical errors in U.S. hospitals. Almost a decade later, The Joint Commission used this statistic to unofficially rank medical errors as the fifth leading cause of death in the United States, ahead of accidents, diabetes, breast cancer, Alzheimer's disease, AIDS, and gunshot wounds (The Joint Commission, 2009). Meanwhile, data was also emerging from The Joint Commission that showed compelling links between **sentinel events** and problems with communication, leadership, and teamwork. (As defined by The Joint Commission, a *sentinel event* "is an unexpected occurrence involving death or serious physical or psychological injury, or the risk thereof" [2013d, para. 1]; sentinel events are discussed in more detail later in this chapter.) In response, patient safety organizations sprang up around the country as problem-solving strategies became a focus for healthcare leaders.

More alarming news came out in the April 2011 issue of the leading healthcare policy journal, *Health Affairs*. Even after more than 10 years of focus on the problem, medical errors, or adverse events, were occurring in about one-third of all hospital admissions and as much as 10 times more than some previous estimates have indicated (Classen et al., 2011). (As defined by the IOM, an **adverse event** "is an injury resulting from a medical intervention, or in other words, it is not due to the underlying medical condition of the patient" [Kohn, Corrigan, & Donaldson, 2000, p. 4].) More recently, a study reported in a 2013 issue of the *Journal of Patient Safety* (James, 2013) found that the true number of premature deaths associated with preventable harm occurring in hospitals was more than 400,000 per year in the United States. This research was conducted by toxicologist John T. James, who became active in patient advocacy following the death of his 19-year-old son, which he maintains was a result of negligence (Allen, 2013). The study was considered controversial, but Harvard pediatrician Lucian Leape, who was involved in the original IOM research and often referred to as the "father of patient safety," has expressed confidence in the findings (Allen, 2013).

The persistence of trouble remains, now 15 years after the release of *To Err Is Human*, as evidenced in comments on error reduction and quality improvement by Ashish Jha, professor of Health Policy and Management at the Harvard School of Public Health. In a testimony before a Senate Subcommittee on Primary Health and Aging hearing in July 2014, Jha commented that "[w]e have not moved the needle in any meaningful, demonstrable way overall. In certain areas, things are better; in certain areas, things are probably worse, but we are not substantially better off compared to where we were [15 years ago]" (More than 1,000 preventable deaths, 2014, 33:35).

PRIMARY ORGANIZATIONS INVOLVED IN PATIENT SAFETY

Although it is hard to know exact numbers because research methods and definitions vary, reporting is not consistent, and types of mistakes differ, there is growing attention to errors in healthcare, and the general consensus among healthcare leaders is that there is much work to be done to make healthcare safer. In response, many leading organizations have gotten involved in efforts to improve patient safety. Each group has a website with vast and varied resources associated with patient safety:

- AHRQ (www.ahrq.gov): The mission of AHRQ is to "produce evidence to make healthcare safer, higher quality, more accessible, equitable, and affordable" (AHRQ, n.d., para. 3).
- Institute for Healthcare Improvement (IHI; www.ihi.org): The IHI is "an independent not-for-profit organization based in Cambridge, Massachusetts, [and] a leading innovator ... in health and healthcare improvement worldwide" (IHI, 2014, para. 1).
- IOM (www.iom.edu): The IOM is "an independent, nonprofit organization that works outside of government to provide unbiased and authoritative advice to decision-makers and the public" (IOM, 2014, para. 1).
- The Joint Commission (www.jointcommission.org): The Joint Commission is an independent, not-for-profit organization that "accredits and certifies more than 20,000 healthcare organizations and programs in the United States. Joint Commission accreditation and certification is recognized nationwide as a symbol of quality that reflects an organization's commitment to meeting certain performance standards" (The Joint Commission, 2013a, para. 1).
- National Patient Safety Foundation (NPSF; www.npsf.org): "A central voice for patient safety since 1997, describes their mission: "NPSF partners with patients and families,

the health care community, and key stakeholders to advance patient safety and health care workforce safety and disseminate strategies to prevent harm." (NPSF, 2015,).

■ QSEN Institute (www.qsen.org): The overall goal of QSEN is to "address the challenge of preparing future nurses with the knowledge, skills, and attitudes (KSAs) necessary to continuously improve the quality and safety of the healthcare systems in which they work" (QSEN Institute, 2014, para. 1).

The Joint Commission, in particular, has been active in obtaining data and reporting on the incidence of serious medical errors, which will be explored next.

Confident Voices

Patricia Ann Bemis, RN, CEN, LHCRM
Online Course Facilitator

A Few Mnemonics for Keeping Communication Orderly and Pertinent

Effective communication is important in all aspects of life. I do not believe that anyone wakes up in the morning and says, "I'm going to communicate ineffectively today." So, if our goal is effective communication—and I assume it is—we must have knowledge of what effective communication is and how to achieve it. As I look back on my schooling, I do not remember a course on effective communication. I do remember a course in journalism that taught me a method that helped me write successful articles for that course: to cover early in the article the who, what, when, where, why, how, and how much.

After graduating and while working as an emergency nurse, I saw patients before they saw the physician. Effectively and concisely communicating the patient's problem to a physician is paramount to the proper diagnosis, treatment, and outcome. I modified the communication tool I learned in my journalism course and used it whenever I discussed a patient with an emergency physician or other staff member. It never failed me. It is as follows: The patient's identity, chief complaint, and history of present illness are developed by interview; then the following information is communicated to the physician:

- **Who:** Identifies the patient by name, age, sex, and lifestyle
- **What:** Explains the symptom(s) that prompted the patient to seek medical advice
- **When:** Tells the time of onset of the symptom(s)
- **Where:** Names the body system or part that is involved and any associated symptoms
- **Why:** Describes any precipitating factors or events
- **How:** Designates how the symptom affects normal function
- **How much:** Labels the severity of the affect as related to normal function

Continued

Confident Voices—cont'd

During my career, I also was certified as an intensive care nurse and worked in the critical care units across the country as a traveling nurse. My communication tool continued to work well, but I needed a different tool to quickly evaluate my patients when they returned from surgery. I developed the following aide-mémoire for receiving a postsurgical patient:

- **A for Awareness:** Evaluate awareness. Talk to the patient.
- **A for Airway:** Assess airway patency and security of mechanical airway.
- **B for Breathing:** Auscultate breath sounds for quality and equality. Monitor pulse oximetry and assess the need for arterial blood gases (ABGs).
- **C for Circulation:** Attach electrocardiogram (ECG) and pressure monitors. Run strips and interpret. Palpate pulses. Assess body temperature, moisture, and color.
- **D for Drugs:** Scrutinize fluids and drugs infusing.
- **D for Dressings:** Inspect dressings for dryness and integrity.
- **D for Drains:** Examine all drains. Connect to suction or gravity; mark or empty containers. Note color, amount, and consistency.
- **D for Diagnostic tests:** Obtain necessary x-ray, ECG, ABGs, and laboratory tests.

This tool works in many situations. Whenever I'm confronted with an emergency patient, I use this quick AABC aide-mémoire to assess the patient. I do the same thing every time I confront a patient, and I am able to intervene quickly if needed or assure myself that the patient is safe:

- **A for Awareness:** I say, "Hi, my name is Pat Bemis. What is your name?" The patient's response will determine awareness.
- **A for Airway:** If the patient responds to my question with clear speech, the airway is patent.
- **B for Breathing:** I look at the patient's overall color and respiratory effort. If the color is pink and the respiratory effort is easy, breathing is adequate and no intervention is needed.
- **C for Circulation:** I note body temperature, moisture, and color by shaking the patient's hand and quickly noting the body temperature, moisture, and color. A finger over the radial pulse determines whether a radial pulse is present and denotes a systolic blood pressure higher than 90.
- **D for Disability:** Evaluation of the patient's posture and handshake gives a quick assessment of debility.

I've learned that not only do these tools help to assess the patient and make appropriate interventions, but they also provide an easy memory of my actions when questioned by a supervisor, physician, or even in court at a later date. In my mind, effective communication needs a few mnemonics to keep it orderly and pertinent and to keep patients safe.

Biography

Patricia Ann Bemis, RN, CEN, LHCRM, is a national speaker, teacher, and author with more than 30 years of experience in the healthcare industry. She is licensed as a healthcare risk manager in the state of Florida and served as president of the National Nurses in Business Association for 15 years. She is the recipient of the Great 100 Nurses Award presented by the Florida Nurses Association and a leader in the field of nurse entrepreneurship and forensic nursing. Her books include *Self-Employed RN: How to Become a Self-Employed RN and/or Business Owner* (2011, National Nurses in Business Association) and *Emergency Nursing Bible: Principles and Practice of Complaint-Based Emergency Nursing*, 5th edition (2010, National Nurses in Business Association).

SENTINEL EVENT STATISTICS

The Joint Commission tracks incidences and types of sentinel events that are voluntarily reported by hospitals, clinics, home care, long-term care facilities, and other healthcare settings that it accredits (The Joint Commission, 2013d). The Joint Commission also investigates and tracks root causes of sentinel events—in other words, the underlying problems or circumstances that led to them. For the purposes of this text, specific sentinel event data are being isolated with the explicit intention of demonstrating links among patient safety, sentinel events, and communication and human behavior. In addition, the statistics discussed offer a somewhat limited view because not all sentinel events are reported to The Joint Commission and not all mistakes result in loss of limb or function, which exclude them from being reported as sentinel events. Data are updated quarterly on The Joint Commission website and include information about the types, practice settings, frequency, and states of origin of sentinel events. The Joint Commission has been tracking data since 1995, which coincides roughly with when awareness of patient safety issues was heightened, and has been providing reports that show trends over time.

A review of the most frequent types of sentinel events accentuates the degree of problems in patient safety and demonstrates the relationships among patient safety, sentinel events, and communication and human behavior. Data from The Joint Commission (2013b) indicate that the most frequent types of sentinel events reviewed in 2011and 2012 were as follows:

1. Unintended retention of a foreign body
2. Wrong site, wrong patient, or wrong procedure
3. Delay in treatment

In 2013, the order changed, but the top three were the same (The Joint Commission, 2013b):

1. Delay in treatment
2. Wrong site, wrong patient, or wrong procedure
3. Unintended retention of a foreign body

One can surmise from this information that it is at least questionable whether efforts to enhance safety in these areas have been effective. To better understand why, examining their underlying causes, or root cause analysis, is necessary.

ROOT CAUSE ANALYSIS

Root cause analysis (RCA) is a process of inquiry and review that is initiated after an error; it seeks to answer the question: "How and why did this error take place?" RCA focuses on processes and systems with the objective of preventing future incidents. There may be more than one root cause involved in any sentinel event, and sometimes there are several; therefore, root causes tend to be grouped in categories and subcategories. Also, there are different models or approaches to RCA and variations in such areas as software, cost, accuracy, depth of review, and facility preference.

When a sentinel event occurs in a hospital, the organization may hire a service to do an RCA. The results can be sent to The Joint Commission along with plans to address the problems identified with processes or systems. Hospitals can also conduct a proactive RCA, which can be done before a new procedure or equipment such as a computer system is implemented or if inconsequential mistakes are noted in current processes in order to prevent sentinel events.

The Joint Commission uses the information to generate reports on the root causes of sentinel events and allows for the viewing of trends over time. In The Joint Commission report, *Sentinel Event Data: Root Causes by Event Type, 2004–2013*, there is a list of 18 commonly identified root cause categories and subcategories (The Joint Commission, 2013c). For a particular type of sentinel event, with information gathered from all reporting agencies, its root causes from 2004 to 2013 are identified. For example, for the sentinel event "unintended retention of a foreign body," the leading root cause category listed is leadership, followed by human factors, and then communication. For "wrong site, wrong patient, wrong procedure" events, the top three root causes noted are, in order, leadership, communication, and human factors. For the sentinel event "delay in treatment," the main root cause is communication, followed by assessment and then human factors; leadership came in fourth. Interestingly, human factors, leadership, and communication show up as the overall leading root cause categories involving all types of events in 2011, 2012, and 2013.

ADDRESSING SENTINEL EVENTS WITH COMMUNICATION

Isolating specific information from the *Sentinel Event Data* report allows for recognizing the critical role of communication and respectful workplace relationships in combating sentinel events. Within the top root causes—human factors, leadership, and communication—and their subcategories, there are some fluid, unpredictable, and tough-to-measure components of communication and human behavior that are directly or indirectly related to them. The subcategories include the following (The Joint Commission, 2013c):

■ Human factors: staffing levels, staffing skill mix, staff orientation, in-service education, competency, assessment, staff supervision, resident supervision,

Confident Voices

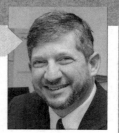

Robert J. Latino, BS, BAM
CEO

Failure to Effectively Communicate: A Root Cause Analysis Perspective

We hear "poor communication" so often related to undesirable outcomes that the term has become somewhat generic in nature. How can we act on poor communication without understanding what causes such miscommunications? This essay highlights key principles of a comprehensive cause-and-effect RCA that are related to discovering underlying causes of miscommunications.

In my work, I use a logic tree diagram and questioning process that leads to explanations about how an undesired outcome could happen. (Students will find a more in-depth review of this process as used in the RCA of the magnetic resonance imaging accident and subsequent death of Michael Colombini [Gilk, Arch, & Latino, 2011].)

As a career investigator, I was involved with a team exploring the decision-making process in arteriovenous fistula (AVF) placement in hemodialysis patients. In one case, a physician team was charted to understand why dialysis patients were choosing catheters and grafts as their primary choice for access versus an AVF, even though AVF was the safest and most preferred access for such patients.

Although more complicated than discussed here, we started out by developing two hypotheses that would explain why patients were not choosing AVF placement:

1. The patient was inappropriate for AVF placement, and/or
2. There was vessel nonpreservation.

For the sake of our case and our focus on poor communication, we are going to follow the first hypothesis by asking, "*How could* the patient be inappropriate for AVF placement?" This leads us to the next hypotheses:

1. The patient refused the AVF placement, and/or
2. It was the physician's decision.

When we continue to drill down in this manner, we will eventually come to decision makers. At the point we reach a decision maker, we change our questioning from "*How could*?" to ask "*Why*?" In other words, why did the decision maker feel the decision made at the time was appropriate?

In our case, we will continue down the path to where the patient is making the decision to not use the AVF option. Why are the patients not using that option?

Continued

Confident Voices—cont'd

One hypothesis developed was that there were patient education issues, and for our purposes we'll pursue how these lead the patient to choose placement options other than an AVF.

At this point, many opinions were expressed that were related to the patient's incompetence or inability to understand the access options. As a lead investigator, my charter is to remain neutral and focus only on the facts. Although the team's expressions were valid hypotheses, they did not express all of the possibilities related to how the patient makes the decision.

I told the team that as a nonclinician, I was closer to the perspective of the patient in such a situation. If I had just been diagnosed with chronic kidney disease, I would initially be in shock. I would have no idea what a fistula was, much less a catheter or graft. So how does a patient learn about these options?

Whenever we educate anyone, it is a form of communication. We need to have a person delivering the message, the content of the message itself, and a person receiving the message. As we explored potential issues related to educational factors, we discovered a variety of possible contributing factors, many of which involve communication:

• The patient educational content was not provided in all the languages needed.
• The patient did not know about the availability of educational content.
• There was inadequate cognitive ability of the patient to understand the message.
• Patient health literacy was less than adequate.
• The educators did not have enough time to properly communicate with the patient.
• The educators were poor teachers.
• Scarce human resources were available for performing such education.
• The educators failed to use available materials for such education.
• The educators were not culturally competent to communicate with some patients.

It is more difficult to look at ourselves as potential contributing factors, yet absolutely necessary in order to promote effective communication.

Why would the educators have poor teaching skills?

• Lack of proper supervisory oversight of such delivered training (no one is observing to see if such education/communication is effective or not)
• Nonexistent training processes and protocols to follow
• Inadequate training processes/practices in place

Oftentimes, education is not a high priority because it is viewed as a "soft" (people) issue. It is hard to demonstrate a return on investment for such issues, so we tend to downplay it. However, we can certainly demonstrate a cost when this

Confident Voices—cont'd

lack of effective communication results in a poor outcome with a claim filed or if a patient is readmitted because of a preventable complication.

I have tried to demonstrate an overview of a logic tree approach to understanding how poor communication affects patient safety. If the causes are properly addressed, they will dramatically improve future communications and therefore the desired outcome.

Reference

Gilk, T., Arch, M., & Latino, R. J. (2011, November/December). MRI safety 10 years later: What can we learn from the accident that killed Michael Colombini? *Patient Safety and Quality Healthcare*. Retrieved from psqh. com/novemberdecember-2011/992-mri-safety-10-years-later?highlight= WyJtcmkiLCJzYWZldHkiLCJtcmkgc2FmZXR5Il0=

Biography

Robert Latino is an internationally recognized expert in the field of RCA and is CEO of Reliability Center, Inc. (www.reliability.com), a 40-year-old Reliability Engineering consulting firm specializing in improving equipment, process, and human reliability. Latino may be contacted at blatino@reliability.com

medical staff credentialing/privileging, medical staff peer review, and other (e.g., rushing, fatigue, distraction, complacency, and bias)

- Leadership: organizational planning, organizational culture, community relations, service availability, priority setting, resource allocation, complaint resolution, leadership collaboration, standardization (e.g., clinical practice guidelines), directing department/services, integration of services, inadequate policies and procedures, noncompliance with policies and procedures, performance improvement, medical staff organization, and nursing leadership
- Communication: oral, written, and electronic, among staff, with and among physicians, with administration, and with patient or family

As black and white as these categories and subcategories seem in written form, many have behavioral components with potential variables or shades of gray to consider. For example, under "human factors," consider the subcategory "staffing levels." Ideal staffing is extremely complicated, and understaffing is an obvious safety risk. Nevertheless, nurses who have the ability to delegate, ask for, offer, and accept help—all communication skills involving self-awareness—can have a positive impact on staffing levels, especially when the organizational culture they work in is responsive to their needs.

Under "leadership," the subcategory "leadership collaboration" very likely involves relationships among nurse managers of a hospital and the chief nursing officer (CNO). Managers must work with the CNO together as a highly functional team; dysfunctional dynamics will create an unhealthy work environment. There must be trust, mutual respect, and effective communication between team members and the CNO.

Inherent in the "communication" category overall as well as in its subcategories is speaking up and listening. Speaking up and listening ineffectively shows up as a contributing cause of a variety of sentinel event types. For instance, "priority setting" (under "leadership") requires an ability to balance organizational or patient needs with one's own availability and respect for the availability of others. Setting limits, negotiating for more resources, and delegating tasks are behaviors that require effective communication that could prevent an error. Many nurses have a hard time setting limits or saying "no," yet doing both is very important. By not doing so, nurses may ignore or postpone priorities, such as monitoring a patient's intravenous pain medication or getting necessary rest. The patient whose pain is well managed is less likely to be anxious and try to get out of bed without assistance and risk falling, and the rested nurse is more alert and less likely to make mistakes.

Further, setting limits requires finding help or, if that help is not available, raising awareness of the need for resources and/or clarifying realistic expectations from patients, families, and leaders. The following scenario illustrates a fluid exchange involving asking for help, setting limits, and delegating: A nurse is in the process of discharging a patient, who has a lot of questions about her discharge medications, when a new admission comes in. She asks another nurse for help: "Can you get started on the new admission while I take some time with her?" Her colleague shakes her head and responds, "I don't have time right now to help you with your new admission, but the unit manager just got back from lunch. I just saw her go into her office." The nurse approaches the unit manager: "Mrs. Holmes has a lot of questions about her discharge medications. Can you get started on the new admission while I take some time with her?" The unit manager offers an alternative solution: "I'd like you to start the admission and get to know him, because you are working this weekend. I'll sit down with Mrs. Holmes and her family to answer her medication questions." If the unit manager is not available to help either, this may indicate to her the need for additional staffing or training in technical skills or time management. An awareness of these issues can be applied to other subcategories under "leadership," including "leadership collaboration," "community relations," "integration of services," and "nursing leadership," as well as the subcategories "staffing levels," "staffing skill mix," and "communication with staff, patients, and families" under the "communication" category.

The previous scenario demonstrates how being aware of and expressing one's own limitations can be crucial for safe care. Although nurses cannot predict when a new admission will come in, where the unit manager might be at any given minute, or how many questions a patient will have about her discharge plan, nurses must always be clear and professional about their needs or limitations, making speaking up and listening effectively a critical function of patient safety and avoiding sentinel events.

As students gain an appreciation for the links between the root causes of sentinel events and communication and behavior, the need to develop emotional intelligence and practice effective and respectful communication will be reinforced.

Consultant Commentary

A few years ago, I was preparing an interactive workshop on communication and assertiveness for a chapter of the Association of Perioperative Registered Nurses (AORN). I asked members of AORN's educational committee to share the most common communication challenges. AORN replied with the following four scenarios:

- Your teammate purposefully holding back information about a surgery to make you look bad in front of the surgeon

- A surgeon yelling that she wants someone in the operating room who "knows what they are doing"
- Purposeful negative discussion about you in the operating room by other team members without including you in the conversation
- A surgeon compromising patient safety by surgical technique (e.g., not wanting to wait for "time-out" or not wanting to wait for "counts" at the end of the procedure, especially when counts are incorrect) and ignoring or becoming angry at requests that he or she consider the information presented

These scenarios reveal layers of interwoven relationship patterns that are fraught with poor communication and dysfunctional behaviors. There may also be a lack of awareness about individual behaviors and their impact on others along with a lack of skill in self-reflection. The complexity of interpersonal dynamics and their ramifications begin to emerge.

Let's consider the scenario of a misplaced surgical sponge. It seems unconscionable that anyone would let this go. In such a case, it might be tempting to jump on the band-wagon and point fingers for what appears to be blatant and outrageous behavior. The obvious solution would surely be to initiate a disciplinary process. But this kind of behavior may be a symptom of bigger problems. Remember, "unintended retention of a foreign body" was the leading type of sentinel event in 2011 and 2012, according to The Joint Commission and based on statistics gathered from operating rooms all over the country.

Before reacting with blaming, let's consider some possible contributing factors that involve the leadership, human factors, and communication:

- The nurse who realizes the sponge is missing has a history of being reprimanded or threatened by a manager or physician, and she perceives her job being put at risk if she speaks up.
- The operating room is on a very tight schedule, and there is a vague yet powerful pressure within the organization to move on to the next patient.
- Another nurse who is a witness is exhausted, and her judgment compromised from work-ing overtime, owing to a combination of emergency surgeries and lack of on-call staff available or willing to come in.
- The surgeon is unaware of how her behaviors affect the team, and she lacks skill in ex-pressing her own needs.

It is very possible to dismiss these factors out of hand as poor excuses for bad behavior. However, without examining these factors, a complex problem is oversimplified, and a knee-jerk solution, such as reprimanding or firing a team member, is decided on, with no effort made to address the underlying issues. Long-term, meaningful solutions must include more in-depth work to develop effective communication and understand the human behaviors associated with it.

CASE STUDY

Caitlyn, a seasoned licensed practical nurse (LPN), is providing care for 20 residents on a 3:00 p.m. to 11:00 p.m. weekend shift in a long-term care facility. There are two licensed nurse assistants (LNAs) working with her, one of whom has just recently completed orientation. A third LNA, who normally floats between this unit and an adjacent one, called in sick, and the supervisor was unable to replace her. The supervisor had promised to help but is kept busy on other units. Throughout the shift, the new LNA has many questions. One of Caitlyn's patients is in respiratory distress and has a temperature of 101°F. She contacts the doctor on call and receives, transcribes, and carries out orders for oxygen, antibiotics, and chest x-ray. Several family members have visited, and Caitlyn has answered their many questions and addressed their concerns. She has also made calls to the physician, pharmacy, and hospice to facilitate a new order for morphine for another patient. There are also quite a few bed alarms and call lights she has to respond to over the course of her shift. She doesn't take any rest or breaks but manages to grab a sandwich. By 10:45 p.m., when the night nurse comes on duty, all the visitors have gone home and most of the residents are in bed. During the narcotics count, the night nurse finds an extra clonazepam and a missing lorazepam. She tells Caitlyn that she made a medication error on a 4:00 p.m. dose. The patient receiving the wrong medication is fine, but Caitlyn feels awful and, not to mention, exhausted.

Discussion Questions

1. What questions would you ask to determine the root cause of this error?
2. What subcategories of the root causes *leadership, human factors,* and/or *communication* might be part of this scenario? Would any of them have possibly contributed to the error? Explain your reasoning.
3. Would the medication error be considered a sentinel event? Why or why not?
4. What suggestions do you have for Caitlyn regarding preventing a future error?

SUMMARY

Gaining a firm grasp on the interrelationship between sentinel events and communication is essential, albeit difficult. As well, raising awareness about the scope of errors may bring up worries and add pressure to clinical experiences. Human beings, even with the best of intentions, are not perfect and have to work hard to prevent mistakes. Fortunately, awareness about human fallibility is on the rise, as evidenced by a pilot project to study the human fallibility in routine tasks currently under way at Boise State University led by nursing instructor Karen Breitkreuz and funded by the ARHQ (Boise State University, 2014). Learning the root causes behind errors is an important step in contributing to safe quality care. This knowledge provides compelling incentive for practicing effective and respectful communication, which in turn creates the foundation for positive work relationships and optimal collaboration, and, in conjunction with more rigorous scientific methods, will bring about needed improvements in patient safety.

Reflection Questions

1. As you begin practice, there will likely be days when you feel rushed, fatigued, and/or overwhelmed with your workload. How do you think that this will affect the care you give? What is your plan for maintaining a high standard of care?

2. Describe a time in a clinical rotation when you made or came close to making a medication error. Explain what happened in terms of following (or not following) the medication administration protocol. Review the subcategories listed in The Joint Commission's sentinel event data and describe how human factors, communication, and/or leadership issues may have contributed.

3. Can you relate to the feeling of wanting to be liked by a physician, nurse, or administrative leader? How will you make sure that any needs for belonging, approval, or a favorable performance evaluation do not interfere with your ability to give constructive feedback to such a person?

References

Agency for Healthcare Research and Quality. (n.d.). About AHRQ. Retrieved from www.ahrq.gov/about/index.html

Allen, M. (2013, September 19). How many die from medical mistakes in U.S. hospitals? *ProPublica*. Retrieved from www.propublica.org/article/how-many-die-from-medical-mistakes-in-us-hospitals

Aspden, P., Corrigan, J. M., Wolcott, J., & Erickson, S. M. (Eds.). (2004). *Patient safety: Achieving a new standard for care*. Washington, DC: National Academies Press.

Boise State University. (2014). Faculty presents pilot study findings at international simulation meeting. Retrieved from hs.boisestate.edu/nursing/2014/04/22/kbreitkreuz-3

Classen, D. C., Resar, R., Griffin, F., Federico, F., Frankel, T., Kimmel, N., ... James, B. C. (2011). "Global trigger tool" shows that adverse events in hospitals may be ten times greater than previously measured. *Health Affairs, 30*(4), 581–589.

Cronenwett, L., Sherwood, G., Barnsteiner, J., Disch, J., Johnson, J., Mitchell, P., . . . Warren, J. (2007). Quality and safety education for nurses. *Nursing Outlook, 55*(3), 122–131.

Edelstein, L. (1943). *The Hippocratic Oath: Text, translation and interpretation*. Baltimore: The John Hopkins Press.

Emanuel, L., Berwick, D., Conway, J., Combes, J., Hatlie, M., Leape, L., ... Walton, M. (2008). What exactly is patient safety? In K. Henriksen, J. B. Battles, M. A. Keyes, & M. L. Gandy (Eds.), *Advances in patient safety: New directions and alternative approaches*, Vol. 1 (pp. 19–36). Rockville, MD: Agency for Healthcare Research and Quality.

Institute for Healthcare Improvement. (2014). About IHI. Retrieved from www.ihi.org/about/pages/default.aspx.

Institute of Medicine. (2001). *Crossing the quality chasm: A new health system for the 21st century*. Washington DC: National Academies Press.

Institute of Medicine. (2014). About the IOM. Retrieved from iom.edu/About-IOM.aspx

James, J. T. (2013). A new, evidence-based estimate of patient harms associated with hospital care. *Journal of Patient Safety, 9*(3), 122–128.

The Joint Commission. (2009). *The Joint Commission guide to improving staff communication* (2nd ed.). Oakbrook Terrace, IL: Joint Commission Resources.

The Joint Commission. (2013a). About The Joint Commission. 2013. Retrieved from www.jointcommission.org/about_us/about_the_joint_commission_main.aspx

The Joint Commission. (2013b). Sentinel event data: General information, 1995–2013. Retrieved from www.joint commission.org/assets/1/18/General_Information_1995-2Q2013.pdf

The Joint Commission. (2013c). Sentinel event data: Root causes by event type, 2004–2013. Retrieved from www.joint commission.org/assets/1/18/Root_Causes_by_Event_Type_2004-2Q2013.pdf

The Joint Commission. (2013d, June 10). Sentinel event policy and procedures. Retrieved from www.jointcommission .org/Sentinel_Event_Policy_and_Procedures

Kohn, L. T., Corrigan, J. M., & Donaldson, M. S. (Eds.). (2000.) *To err is human: Building a safer health system*. Washington, DC: National Academies Press.

More than 1,000 preventable deaths a day is too many: The need to improve patient safety. Hearing before the Subcommittee of the Committee on Health, Education, Labor, and Pensions, Senate, 113th Senate. (2014.) Testimony of Ashish Jha. Retrieved from www.help.senate.gov/hearings/hearing/?id=478e8a35-5056-a032-52f8-a65f8bd0e5ef

National Patient Safety Foundation. (2015.) About us. Retrieved from http://www.npsf.org/?page=aboutus .

Nightingale, F. (1859). *Notes on hospitals*. London: John W. Parker and Sons.

Quality and Safety Education for Nurses Institute. (2014). Project overview. Retrieved from qsen.org/about-qsen/project-overview

Patient Experience

Healthcare professionals often become involved in patients' lives at times when they are vulnerable emotionally and/or physically. Nursing is a career of service that requires an understanding of therapeutic relationships and an appreciation of patient experience. Whereas nurses choose their profession, patients end up in the healthcare system much of the time for reasons beyond their control, such as unexpected injuries and chronic diseases. More than a job, the profession of nursing carries with it a privilege of caring for others during such times and a responsibility to use specialized knowledge, skills, and attitudes (KSAs) to contribute to patients' well-being. Nurses play many vital roles—coach, teacher, and counselor—and they must be able to communicate effectively and respectfully with their patients, who have a wide range of expectations, needs, worries, abilities, resources, and desires. Nurses must understand and be responsive to patients who have varied ability to participate in their own care, while recognizing there is an overall shift in healthcare toward collaborative practice and patient empowerment.

This chapter explores the application of communication skills to therapeutic relationships and for optimizing the patient experience and collaborative practice. Students will be introduced to motivational interviewing as a technique for empowering patients. Finally, students will learn about the Hospital Consumer Assessment of Healthcare Providers and Systems (HCAHPS) survey tool used for measuring patient experience.

THERAPEUTIC RELATIONSHIPS

A **therapeutic relationship** is defined as "a professional, interpersonal alliance in which the nurse and client join together for a defined period to achieve health-related treatment goals" (Arnold & Boggs, 2011, p. 83). This definition can serve as a guidepost when questionable boundaries arise in professional relationships and acts as reminder that the goal of the therapeutic relationship is the health and healing of the client. While the Health Insurance Portability and Accountability Privacy Act of 1996 (HIPAA) regulations provide a legal structure that protects privacy and confidentiality of patient information (U.S. Department of Health and Human Services, n.d.), nurses also must develop good judgment about what is appropriate sharing of information for purposes of developing therapeutic relationships. Understanding elements of dependency and vulnerability will help students navigate complicated relationship boundaries and develop their judgment.

Dependence and Vulnerability

The assessment of a patient's physical abilities and need for physical care is often referred to as **dependency**, which can range from totally dependent to independent. Dependency is not just physical; it can include emotional, educational, and other needs described in Maslow's hierarchy of needs.

Any time a person must rely on another, there is an implicit or explicit dependence inherent in the relationship: Passengers on planes are dependent on pilots and flight attendants, car owners are dependent on mechanics, and patients are dependent on healthcare workers. In addition to being sick or injured, patients in the healthcare system are often frightened, anxious, and overwhelmed. The environment is foreign and noisy. Their personal space is extremely compromised as they are poked and prodded for assessments, diagnostic tests, and treatments. If hospitalized overnight, they are sleeping in a bed that is not theirs and may be sharing a room with a complete stranger. Whether the health issue is temporary or life changing, feelings of **vulnerability** and loss of control are quite understandable.

This dependency and vulnerability result in an interesting power dynamic in healthcare as professionals providing specialized care have expertise that patients and families need, want, and may even be somewhat desperate for. Professionals know how the healthcare facility works, where things are, and what the acronyms mean, and they may know more about what is going on for the patient with regard to his or her health than the patient or family does. Nurses can relieve pain, answer questions, provide education, or contact the physician, which puts them in a privileged role with a lot of power over the patient experience. To be worthy of such power, nurses are responsible for completing the necessary tasks that relate to scope of practice, standard of care, continuing education, and licensing. Such power is associated with a commitment to service and must never be abused or taken lightly. The behavioral approach to communication is consistent with developing therapeutic relationships and ensuring respectful uses of power.

Therapeutic Communication

Therapeutic communication is essentially the application of assertiveness and listening skills used in the course of helping patients reach their health-related goals, which has to some extent already been discussed. Communication skills and emotional intelligence (discussed in Part I) are necessary to obtain important information for the care plan and to build a trusting relationship, both of which will contribute to safe, quality care. Because there are important and sometimes confusing professional boundaries that must be considered in the context of therapeutic relationships, the topic warrants further discussion.

Confident Voices

Martine Ehrenclou, MA
Author and Healthcare Advocate

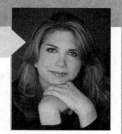

My Empathic Nurse and an Almost Unbearable Night

By the time I was admitted into Cedars-Sinai Medical Center, I was more than ready for surgery. I'd had acute, lower abdominal pain for the past 18 months and had seen 12 physicians to find an accurate diagnosis and treatment plan. The surgeon, a hernia specialist, was my last hope. She'd diagnosed an inguinal hernia and a muscle tear at my C-section site, both with nerves through the holes.

By the time I met Sheila, my RN for the night, I was recovering from a 3-hour surgery, exhausted, and worried about its success. The surgeon's words looped in my head. "I hope this is successful. I can't be sure...."

Dressed in powder-blue scrubs, Sheila greeted me with a warm smile and asked how I was feeling.

"I'm okay," I said, managing a smile.

While checking my IV, vitals, and incisions, Sheila chatted with me for a few minutes as I described what I'd been through over the last 18 months of 10 misdiagnoses, 15 procedures and tests, 22 medications, and more.

"Not one doctor could figure it out," I said.

"You should have seen a nurse," she said, and we both laughed. I didn't go into the bladder installations, steroid injections into my pelvic nerves, the catheterizations, the full year on antibiotics for a diagnosis I never had, and more.

"I just hope this does it."

Sheila placed her hand on my arm. "You've been through it, haven't you?" But it wasn't a question. It was a show of empathy, sincere and from the heart.

I nodded, fighting tears.

After pouring water into a plastic cup, Sheila wrapped my hand around it and asked me to drink. "Want to try to use the restroom?" She explained the importance of emptying my bladder after abdominal surgery.

"I tried before but no luck."

Sheila was a little firmer this time. "I need you to try again. We don't want to catheterize you."

Adrenalin lit my heart. I could not face another catheter. Not now. Not after the urologists with their catheters, the gynecologists with their instruments. My breath now had a life of its own.

"It's okay, sweetie, no rush. We have time. Let's just try." Sheila led me to the bathroom, her arm across my back.

Continued

Confident Voices—cont'd

A few minutes passed inside. I opened the bathroom door to face her. "Can't do it."

We settled into a conversation about her job as a nurse, about mine as a writer. I mentioned that I had interviewed more than 100 nurses for my first book and understood just how hard but rewarding the life of a nurse could be. She then mentioned that she danced every week to relieve stress.

I perked up. "You dance? What kind?"

"Hip hop."

"Me too!"

If Sheila was skeptical about a 50-year-old-white woman taking hip hop classes, she didn't show it. We launched into a conversation about our mutual love of contemporary gospel music, R&B, and dance.

Sheila filled the cup with more water. "Want to try again?"

"I'm not sure I can."

She must have sensed my worry. "I have some tricks to help." She held out her hand to me. I grasped it, and she led me into the bathroom and turned on the faucet. "Sometimes that helps. I'll wait here. You go on in."

The water poured into the sink. Still nothing.

She handed me a small pan of water. "Put your hand in and give it a try."

I plunged my fingers into the warm water. My bladder felt numb.

Sheila led me back to bed. "Sometimes it just takes a while."

The evening faded into night, and the hospital halls grew quiet, with the exception of a few beeps and whirs of machines. I couldn't sleep.

Sheila poked her head in. "You up for company?"

I nodded.

We talked about our favorite artists—Smokie Norful, J. Moss, Deitrick Haddon, and others. She then asked the dreaded question about using the restroom. "We have about 30 minutes left. I don't want to have to catheterize you."

After easing out of bed, I went in and sat for a while. I then heard Sheila singing softly outside the door, a Mahalia Jackson song. I forgot about everything except her lovely voice, that song.

And before I knew it, my bladder relaxed.

Sheila was almost as relieved as I was. Rubbing my back, she said, "Get some rest now."

The surgery was a complete success and relieved me of all pain. I wrote Sheila a thank-you card, expressing my gratitude for her help and letting her know just how special she was as a nurse and as a person. Her empathy and kindness had made a tough night so much more bearable.

Confident Voices—cont'd

Biography

Martine Ehrenclou, MA, is an award-winning author, healthcare advocate, and speaker. She is the author of *The Take-Charge Patient: How You Can Get the Best Medical Care* (2012, Lemon Grove Press) and *Critical Conditions: The Essential Hospital Guide to Get Your Loved One Out Alive* (2008, Lemon Grove Press). Ehrenclou lectures and publishes articles and blogs on the topics of patient empowerment, patient engagement, patient safety, and other aspects of patient-centered care. She has a master's degree in psychology from Pepperdine University and a certificate in patient advocacy from UCLA. Visit her at www.thetakechargepatient.com and www.criticalconditions.com

At times, communication between nurses and patients crosses a professional boundary into a more personal or social realm than may be appropriate. Intuiting what is and is not appropriate is important for nurses, which can be done by staying true to the therapeutic goal and applying communication skills from Part I. Consider the following scenario: A rehab nurse is caring for a patient who has a hand injury. They discover during the admission assessment that they both are avid guitar players. Some therapeutic communication may involve an exchange about popular guitar players, giving the nurse the opportunity to share a little about himself and also show that he feels some empathy for this patient regarding possible limitations posed by the hand injury. However, this nurse must also be mindful of time spent chatting because it might be perceived by the patient as an invitation for a more social relationship, and it also might compromise time needed to care for other patients. It is always a judgment call, so nurses should ask themselves, "Is this conversation necessary and appropriate for the therapeutic relationship I have with this patient?" Going one step further, it would be inappropriate for this RN to plan an outside event with this patient to hear their favorite local guitarist because that is an obvious foray into a social relationship. However, if this nurse meets the patient by accident at a concert 6 months later and the therapeutic relationship has ended, sharing time enjoying music can be done in a healthy and mutual manner. At this point, the nurse and former patient should discuss any residual dependence (discussed more shortly) that the patient might feel or any therapeutic responsibility that the nurse might have.

Here is another scenario that illustrates the importance of good judgment and effective communication in a therapeutic relationship: In a conversation about her treatment plan, a patient mentions to her nurse that she might be interested in getting a second opinion regarding her planned surgery. The nurse senses that the issue is about the patient being scared and perhaps not understanding everything about the surgery. The nurse encourages the patient to express her concerns to the physician in an attempt to empower the patient as well as promote the therapeutic relationship between them and also between the physician and the patient: "I'd really like to share your request with Dr. Pyne, but I'm betting you can do it. What are your thoughts?" If the nurse instead had gone right to the doctor without discussing it with the patient, the patient may have been angry about the nurse doing so without consulting her and the doctor might have felt challenged by the nurse's assumptions. In both circumstances, the therapeutic relationships between nurse and patient and between doctor and patient would be weakened. While the nurse may think she is being helpful by sharing the communication with the doctor, she should be more self-aware about keeping the goal of the therapeutic relationship in mind and recognizing opportunities for empowering the patient. The nurse must also be careful not to withhold information from the physician that may affect treatment or diagnosis even when the patient expresses concerns about it. "It sounds like you are feeling embarrassed about skipping your blood pressure medication and are worried about Dr. Jone's reaction, is that right? She really needs to know so that she can make the best decision about changing your medication, and it would be wrong for me to keep that from her. She's on her way to see you, would it help if I stayed while you tell her?"

Effective therapeutic communication also includes awareness of language appropriateness for age, culture, education, and personal preference. Some general guidelines, such as avoiding use of medical jargon, using simpler terms for children, and talking louder to a geriatric population, are worthwhile to follow. Students should become familiar with any population they are providing care for and always take the time to listen to and learn about each individual patient because the communication process is the path to developing a therapeutic relationship.

PATIENT EXPERIENCE

Patient experience is a newer term in healthcare that is inherent in therapeutic relationships but emphasizes the patient's perspective. Patient experience has been a growing focus of patient advocates and healthcare leaders, in part as a response to alarming and more visible concerns about patient safety (discussed in Chapter 5) and in part as an effort to increase the presence of patient voices in the bigger healthcare picture. The Beryl Institute, an independent global community of practice focusing on improving patient experience, defines patient experience as "the sum of all interactions, shaped by an organization's culture, that influence patient perceptions across the continuum of care" (n.d., para. 1). The inclusion of the terms *interactions*, *culture*, and *perceptions* suggests very powerful associations with communication skills and practices of the healthcare team. Just as nurses are encouraged to use the behavioral approach to communication in developing the therapeutic relationship, they can also use the concepts to optimize patient experience.

A major aspect of the patient experience movement is **patient empowerment**. In her book, *The Take-Charge Patient: How You Can Get the Best Medical Care*, author and leader in patient empowerment, Martine Ehrenclou (2012) emphasizes active patient involvement and accountability by encouraging communication with the healthcare team. Ehrenclou teaches patients how to navigate the complex healthcare system, ask questions, research health issues, and prepare for encounters with healthcare professionals. More and more patients are taking an active role in their care. This is an exciting trend, and nurses must be able to work collaboratively with patients and families who have a continuum of knowledge and increased interest in being active partners. With the huge amount of information and technology available to patients, and with their vested interest in particular diagnoses, some patients may be extremely well informed about their healthcare needs, risks, and options.

Communicating for Optimal Patient Experience

As discussed in Chapter 3, listening respectfully to patients in every interaction should be a priority for nurses. It will help patients to feel heard, build trusting therapeutic relationships, improve patient experience scores, and help patients to become empowered. Questions that set a tone of openness and show interest in a patient's experience include the following:

- Do you have any concerns about tomorrow's MRI?
- I know the admission process can seem like we're trying to fit you in a bunch of little boxes. Are there any questions or worries you have about what happens next?

Consultant Commentary

As a consultant and author, I am an advocate for teaching nurses to be assertive for themselves as well as their patients. I believe therapeutic relationships can be a driving force in shifting the power dynamics in healthcare. In theory, there has always been a focus on the therapeutic relationship, but it now has additional significance with the current focus in healthcare for professionals and consumers to be more collaborative members. Collaborative practice calls on us to shift away from old power dynamics in which physicians have had too much power and nurses, other healthcare professionals, and patients have not had enough. These power dynamics have influenced interprofessional communication and therapeutic relationships in ways that have insidiously interfered with collaboration. Situations in which nurses were afraid to challenge physicians, physicians refused to be challenged, and patients assumed doctors and nurses knew more about their needs than they did have had a counterproductive influence on therapeutic communication. In a survey on behavior in which more than 2,100 doctors and nurses responded, Carrie Johnson (2009) describes examples of reported behaviors, including the following:

- *Tools and other objects being flung across the operating room*
- *Physicians groping nurses and technicians as they tried to perform their jobs*
- *Personal grudges interfering with patient care*
- *Accusations of incompetence or negligence in front of patients and their families*

These examples show how aggressive and passive-aggressive behaviors manifest among healthcare professionals who lack emotional intelligence and disregard the therapeutic relationship. Fears, insecurities, and acceptance of inappropriate behaviors inform interactions and keep us from providing safe, quality care. Nurses who feel a sense of power and security when they are admired by colleagues, physicians, and/or patients must learn to be accountable for bringing their expertise to the table regardless of whether others esteem them. Doctors or other leaders who feel they must always be in control of everything must learn how to collaborate and trust others. All healthcare professionals must work to create environments in which patients are encouraged to speak up and participate with their care while at same time honoring patients who are not ready or able to. This change of course is not going to happen in an instant. However, nursing students who are aware of how they feel, develop self-confidence, and express respect for their peers and instructors, even in the midst of conflict, will play an important role in the shift toward collaborative practice.

- You look upset about the breakfast tray, and I've noticed you haven't been eating. Can you tell me what's on your mind?

When these questions are preceded by validation and empathy, it tells patients that they matter to the people taking care of them. This is worth the time it takes. One way to show empathy is by assessing the patient in a compassionate and inclusionary way. This could be as simple as holding a handheld digital thermometer so that both patient and nurse can see the temperature; this allows the patient to feel included in the process as opposed to being an object of it. Although not all patients will be interested in knowing their temperature or even be able to understand all clinical implications, including them is a great way to find out their levels of interests and knowledge as well as to nurture the evolution of both. Further, the nurse who looks for opportunities to involve patients in their care will demonstrate respect for and interest in the patient's experience.

Another way to involve patients is to ask questions that invite them to participate while honoring their perspective (e.g., "What does this hospitalization feel like to you?" or "Would you like to know what your blood pressure is?"). Optimizing patient experience and independence should be underlying goals for healthcare professionals. Because patients have a range of abilities, desires, and needs, respectful listening and encouragement of assertiveness by nurses are critical.

Part of communicating for optimal patient experience is not only asking questions but also inviting patients to ask questions in a nonthreatening manner. For example, a nurse might say, "Patients are often anxious about surgery and sometimes afraid to ask questions. I want you to know that I'm here to answer any questions you have." This approach infers to the patient that anxiety and fears around asking questions are normal. If this nurse then sits with the patient for a minute, there is a good chance that the patient will believe the nurse is sincere in her offer. This is reassuring to patients, values any concerns they have, and encourages patients to speak up. A nurse who offers to answer questions while racing out the door is not likely to reassure or empower patients because the verbal message is contradicted by the nonverbal message.

When encouraging patients to ask questions, nurses need to be respectful in their answers, keep the therapeutic relationship in mind, and avoid answering defensively. Let's consider a common patient concern, hand washing, or really the lack of, which is an incessant problem in healthcare and is associated with serious hospital acquired infections. With the issue getting more media attention, patients are more likely to notice whether nurses and others wash their hands at appropriate times. However, they may worry that asking or reminding healthcare professionals may jeopardize their relationship with them and, subsequently, negatively impact the care they receive. And, indeed, some healthcare professionals may respond defensively to a patient questioning them about such an obvious and important step in patient care or possibly feel frustrated with time pressures or lack of resources, such as soap and paper towels, that support the process. Instead of getting defensive, nurses should instead express appreciation of the reminder: "You are right! Thank you for the reminder. Since there's no soap at this sink, I was actually going to step out to wash my hands next door and let the manager know we need soap so we'll be ready next time." Notice how this statement is not threatening or defensive, ensures proper procedure, creates an opportunity for the manager to address the underlying problem (i.e., making sure soap is available), and, most important, gives credence to the patient's concern, which may encourage the patient to speak up again. Nurses need to be careful about not making such issues problems for patients while at the same time being honest and seeking avenues to explore concerns.

Although defensiveness is generally an inappropriate reaction to patient questions, reflecting on such answers later and discussing feelings with colleagues and/or management may offer rich rewards. For example, investigating defensiveness may raise awareness about problems such as understaffing, excessive workloads, training needs, or even stocking issues (e.g., soap and paper towels), all of which will affect patient experience.

HCAHPS Survey

As students develop their communication skills to improve patient experience, they should also be aware of how patient feedback is being used to improve care. Historically, many facilities track patient feedback to find ways of improving customer service or increasing revenue via sales and marketing, and for quality control purposes. More recently, because of the shift of power dynamics in the healthcare landscape, patient experience is now ranked in patient surveys. The Centers for Medicare and Medicaid Services (CMS), in conjunction with the Agency for Healthcare Research and Quality, has worked in the last decade to standardize feedback from patients and create ways for consumers to compare service from different hospitals. Ensuring positive or at least optimal patient experience has become a compelling initiative for many hospitals. In theory, at least, publicizing data aids consumers in making informed healthcare decisions and provides incentives for hospitals to improve quality. To address this theory, in 2006, CMS (2013a) developed the HCAHPS survey to collect feedback from patients in order to standardize measures across the country, provide quality improvement incentives, and increase transparency and public accountability. The survey is administered to random samples of adult patients who have been hospitalized in medical, surgical, and maternity departments, within 48 hours to 6 weeks of their stay. With a requirement of 300 completed surveys over four calendar quarters, hospitals are required to survey patients monthly using CMS-approved survey vendors. Alternatively, they can seek approval from CMS to do their own surveys and have the option of adding additional questions after the core HCAHPS items.

The HCAHPS survey (CMS, 2013b) is composed of 32 items, 18 of which encompass critical aspects of the hospital experience, including communication with doctors, communication with nurses, responsiveness of hospital staff, cleanliness of the hospital environment, quietness of the hospital environment, pain management, communication about medicines, discharge information, overall rating of the hospital, and recommendation of the hospital. Of these 18 items, the 14 that follow are directly related to communication and emotional intelligence (CMS, 2013b):

- During this hospital stay, how often did nurses treat you with courtesy and respect? (p. 1)
- During this hospital stay, how often did nurses listen carefully to you? (p. 1)
- During this hospital stay, how often did nurses explain things in a way you could understand? (p. 1)
- During this hospital stay, how often did doctors treat you with courtesy and respect? (p. 2)
- During this hospital stay, how often did doctors listen carefully to you? (p. 2)
- During this hospital stay, how often did doctors explain things in a way you could understand? (p. 2)
- During this hospital stay, how often was the area around your room quiet at night? (p. 2)
- Before giving you any new medicine, how often did hospital staff tell you what the medicine was for? (p. 3)
- Before giving you any new medicine, how often did hospital staff describe possible side effects in a way you could understand? (p. 3)
- During this hospital stay, did doctors, nurses, or other hospital staff talk with you about whether you would have the help you needed when you left the hospital? (p. 3)
- During this hospital stay, did you get information in writing about what symptoms or health problems to look out for after you left the hospital? (p. 3)
- During this hospital stay, staff took my preferences and those of my family or caregiver into account in deciding what my healthcare needs would be when I left. (p. 10)
- When I left the hospital, I had a good understanding of the things I was responsible for in managing my health. (p. 10)
- When I left the hospital, I clearly understood the purpose for taking each of my medications. (p. 10)

The use of verbs such as *listen, explain, understand,* and *describe* encourage survey takers to consider the role interpersonal communication played in their hospital stay.

Respecting feedback to the survey is important and can contribute to improved care. However, because many people enter the healthcare system because they have to, not because they want to (the experience of which, for some, may involve much tragedy and loss), survey scores may reflect anger and grief that are not accurate interpretations of the hospital experience. In the same vein, patients and families may seek to have control in any way possible when loss of control in other parts of their life is threatened. Negative feedback needs to be weighed carefully and objectively in order to ensure valid opinions that could help to create a better patient experience are used while being mindful that some responses may include feelings projecting anger or grief that are unfairly directed at staff or the organization.

Although the survey gives patients the opportunity to air grievances and voice legitimate complaints, not all feedback is critical in nature. In fact, many patients feel great relief and deep appreciation after an extended stay in the hospital, and the survey provides them with an opportunity to express gratitude. Reading positive feedback can prove beneficial to healthcare professionals, in that it can balance the day-to-day stress that contributes to burnout with reminders about some core reasons they chose to pursue a career in healthcare.

Since the development of the HCAHPS survey, CMS reimbursement rates have become tied to hospital compliance in collecting and reporting data. Survey results are also tabulated and available to the public on the Hospital Compare website (www.medicare.gov/hospitalcompare/search.html) so that consumers can see how Medicare-certified hospitals rate in respect to patient experience and additional data, such as timeliness and effectiveness of care, readmission rates, use of medical imaging, and number of Medicare patients and Medicare payments. If consumers go to the Hospital Compare website and enter their zip code, they can select three hospitals in their area at one time to obtain data.

As healthcare professionals become more adept at taking constructive feedback and consumers more adept at offering it, it is likely that survey tools such as the HCAHPS survey will have a better chance at creating positive change.

Confident Voices

Lynn McVey, MS
CEO

A CEO's View of Care Coordination From the Inside

Unfortunately, I had an insider's view of the care coordination we deliver in our healthcare system early in 2014. Fortunately, I am the acting CEO of a community hospital, so I was able 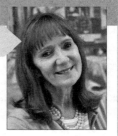 to advocate for my 92-year-old dad as he received critical care at three different hospitals within 3 days for life-saving interventions. However, I firmly believe it was only because I have worked in all three hospitals and my cell phone contains a magical and priceless list of healthcare contacts. I do not believe my dad would be alive today if I wasn't there, 24/7, with my clinical knowledge base and contacts.

More recently, I did the same for a best friend needing a series of abdominal surgeries. Even though he lives in a different state, I convinced him to travel to my hospital. I told him how dangerous hospitals are and that he would be in a much safer environment with me as an insider.

Confident Voices—cont'd

During his surgery, I played "undercover boss" and snuck in the back door of his OR. Dressed in a mask, hat, and scrubs, nobody knew it was me. I was actually surprised to witness well-oiled care coordination, even when an unexpected event occurred and staff had to scramble.

My friend and my dad both provided me with the opportunity to see what's right and what's wrong with our hospitals. For example, I intercepted two medical errors during my father's admission. If I wasn't there to question them, he would have had an unnecessary x-ray and laboratory test. In my friend's case, at 2:30 a.m. the night after his surgery, he waited 35 minutes for the call bell to be answered. His room was in a remote section, and luckily his needs weren't urgent, but it frightened him. It made me question why our postoperative patients aren't near the nurses' station.

Preventable medical errors are rampant. Care coordination is an oxymoron. Over the years when money was in abundance, we created an overspecialized, fragmented, jigsaw of a process. Let's look at medical imaging as one example. We have specialized the imaging technologists into diagnostic techs, CT techs, MRI techs, nuclear techs, PET techs, mammography techs, and ultrasound techs. Ultrasound techs are specialized even further into vascular techs, obstetric and gynecological ultrasound techs, echocardiography techs, and neurosonography techs. Overspecialized healthcare providers are part of the problem today.

On a whim, I counted the number of providers who visited my dad and my friend: 28 different specialists came into the room every day. They asked the same questions. They asked different questions. They performed different tests, gave different medications, and unfortunately, delivered different information: "Don't lift more than 10 pounds" versus "Don't lift more than 50 pounds" is a 40-pound difference!

After being on the inside of these two admissions, my vision is for a *1:1 nurse/ advocate to in-patient ratio*—in other words, one nurse who will navigate care coordination during a patient's hospitalization. As much as possible, the same nurse would draw blood, obtain vitals, give medications, order meals, recite patient allergies, repeat patient history to anyone who asks, transport the patient to radiology and back again, and educate and develop the discharge plan. This one nurse, by this close association, could advocate and protect the patient from errors.

I haven't calculated the financial impact, and not every patient needs this 1:1 ratio, but for the elderly, alone, and critical patients, I wonder how many expensive errors, unnecessary tests, infections, falls, extended days, and preventable deaths could be avoided by this 1:1 approach. It is crystal clear to me that we have built a healthcare system that is too complex to fix. If any of us had the opportunity to rebuild healthcare from scratch, it would never look like it does today.

Continued

Confident Voices—cont'd

For everyone in the healthcare industry who has direct patient responsibilities, please engage and connect with your patients. Conversation is the action in which patients perceive competence. Conversation means speaking to the patient, listening while the patient responds, replying relevant to their response, listening to their response again, and repeating. Conversation is a two-way information exchange. Unfortunately, what I witnessed was mostly one-way information delivered to the patient with the assumption that the patient understood.

"Communication" complaints are an outlier on our patient satisfaction surveys: 26% of our complaints identify poor, rushed, confusing, and inadequate communication as a patient dissatisfier. We've drilled this down further to find that the residents' communication is the source of many complaints. I will personally present our expectations to the residents on a routine basis. Our expectation is that before leaving the patient's room, they are to obtain eye contact with the patient and ask three questions, "Is there anything I need to explain further to you?" "What questions do you have for me? and "What can I do for you before I leave your room?" Because improving communication is a hospital-wide issue, all nursing and nonnursing staff will be educated regarding these three questions. Keeping every patient safe is an enormous task—and it is your job.

Biography

Lynn McVey is acting president and CEO of Meadowlands Hospital Medical Center in Secaucus, New Jersey. Her subject matter expertise is evidence-based management. This "Data Diva" is passionate about healthcare and believes "traditional" healthcare management is no longer a viable model to improve the mess we're in today. She has multiple publications, and recently, she and her partners authored *The Book on Evidence Based Management in Healthcare: The Game Changer* (2012, Imaging Fusion). She is also a popular guest blogger for Fierce Healthcare (www.fiercehealthcare.com).

MOTIVATIONAL INTERVIEWING

Motivational interviewing is a collaborative approach to communicating with patients that is especially effective in supporting behavioral changes that contribute to healthier lifestyles. The technique consequently strengthens therapeutic relationships and improves the patient experience. Pioneered in the 1980s and developed by William Miller and Stephen Rollnick (2013), motivational interviewing, which is covered by many resources that focus on training, is especially helpful with health-related behaviors involving substance abuse, smoking cessation, diet, and exercise habits. Nurses have frequent opportunities to counsel patients on such topics and have a responsibility to address them in as effective a manner as possible. Although not designed to be a motivational interviewing training guide, this book covers similar principles because the overall premise of respectful and empowering communication is a common theme. The technique is effectively demonstrated in two short YouTube videos, "The Ineffective Physician: Non-Motivational Approach" (www.youtube.com/watch?v=80XyNE89eCs) and "The Effective Physician Motivational Interviewing Demonstration" (www.youtube.com/watch?v=DDeXwF8Ff3E).

There are some basic dos and don'ts when discussing behavioral changes that are common in motivational interviewing strategies. *Do practice reflective listening* and look for opportunities to empathize and validate the patient's perspective: "It sounds like you've been trying to exercise more, but find it hard to fit in with your work and family life. Working two jobs to make ends meet must be very stressful, and I can understand why exercising may be the last thing you want to add to your schedule."

Do look for opportunities to accentuate current or past positive efforts with a focus on the patient's own incentive for change: "It sounds like you were eating healthier foods during your pregnancy last year. Can you say more about that?" An incentive for healthy eating while pregnant may translate into role modeling or being around longer for one's children. It is important to let patients discover their own motivation; the nurse's role is to pay close attention, be curious, and help make connections: "It sounds like being pregnant helped you to prioritize eating and exercise. Is that right? Do you think there may be more ways that your son might benefit from your eating and exercise practices?"

Don't scold, lecture, judge, accuse, or assume to know what the patient should do. Providing education that is cloaked with any of these attitudes is not likely to teach or inspire patients to change behavior. Most people already have some level of awareness about poor health behaviors, so they may gain the most benefit from learning specifics that healthcare professionals have to offer. Regardless, if they feel judged or accused, they are not likely to be receptive to learning. So avoid accusatory questions that may invoke a defensive response, such as "Are you eating a lot of junk food?" or "Why haven't you become familiar with the side effects of this medication?"

CASE STUDY

Curran is a staff RN who works 3:00 p.m. to 11:00 p.m. on an orthopedic floor in a teaching hospital. Toward the end of his shift, he receives a call from the emergency department that they are sending up an elderly woman who has suffered a fracture of her left arm; she is scheduled for surgery the next day. Curran goes to the emergency room, where a nurse introduces him to Mrs. Caswell. She is lying on a gurney, and Curran notices that although she's awake, she appears groggy and a bit anxious. The emergency department nurse brings Curran up to date on the situation: The 91-year-old patient came here by ambulance following a fall at home. She has a comminuted fracture of the left humerus and has been scheduled for an open reduction and internal fixation in the morning. Her labs are good. She was medicated with 5 mg of MSO_4 at 9:00 p.m. with good effect. She has signed consents for surgery. Her arm is in a sling, and she is to minimize movement. Curran smiles at Mrs. Caswell and asks if she has any family with her. She shakes her head and tells Curran she has lived alone with her cat Lucy since her husband passed away 2 years earlier. According to her records, she has never been hospitalized and has never had any surgeries, although she accompanied her late husband through multiple admissions.

Discussion Questions

1. Based on the information he has learned so far, what fears or worries might Curran expect Mrs. Caswell to have regarding her impending surgery?

2. What communication strategies might Curran use to help Mrs. Caswell express her concerns?

3. What opportunities might there be to build a therapeutic relationship with this patient? What are some things Curran could say to alleviate some of Mrs. Caswell's fears?

SUMMARY

Healthy, effective therapeutic relationships and optimal patient experience require excellent communication skills and emotional intelligence. Consumers have varying healthcare needs, and preferences differ significantly from person to person. Even patients who have an identical diagnosis are likely to have different support systems, medical knowledge, and fears. Professionals who are able to listen both to assess clinical status and to understand a patient's concerns will contribute to optimal patient experiences. Nurses must put the pen down for a few minutes to show that they are listening to the people who come to them for care. Staying in touch with true curiosity and empathy are practices that build and maintain therapeutic relationships.

Reflection Questions

1. Consider a patient whom you have cared for during a recent clinical experience. How would you describe the therapeutic relationship you had with him or her? What communication strategies did you use or could you have used to enhance the relationship? How do you think this patient might have answered questions on the HCAHPS survey?

2. Have you ever had or can you imagine being tempted to have a more social relationship with one of your patients? Describe how this could interfere with the therapeutic relationship you are trying to develop.

3. Imagine what it might be like to suddenly find yourself in the hospital. What do you think an optimal patient experience would include?

References

Arnold, E. C., & Boggs, K. U. (2011). *Interpersonal relationships: Professional communication skills for nurses* (6th ed., p. 83). St. Louis: Elsevier Saunders.

The Beryl Institute. (n.d.). Retrieved from www.theberylinstitute.org

Centers for Medicare and Medicaid Services. (2013a). HCAHPS fact sheet. Retrieved from www.hcahpsonline.org/files/August_2013_HCAHPS_Fact_Sheet3.pdf

Centers for Medicare and Medicaid Services. (2013b). HCAHPS survey. Retrieved from www.hcahpsonline.org/files/HCAHPS%20V8.0%20Appendix%20A%20-%20HCAHPS%20Mail%20Survey%20Materials%20%28English%29%20March%202013.pdf

Ehrenclou, M. (2012). *The take-charge patient: How you can get the best medical care.* Santa Monica, CA: Lemon Grove Press.

Johnson, C. (2009). Bad blood: Doctor-nurse behavior problems impact patient care. *Physician Executive Journal, 35*(6), 6–11. Retrieved from www.ache.org/policy/doctornursebehavior.pdf

Miller, W. R., & Rollnick, S. (2013). *Motivational interviewing: Helping people change* (3rd ed.). New York: The Guilford Press.

U.S. Department of Health and Human Services. (n.d.). HIPAA administrative simplification statute and rules. Retrieved from www.hhs.gov/ocr/privacy/hipaa/administrative/index.html

CHAPTER 7

Respectful Workplaces

- Discuss types of disrespectful and abusive behavior in the workplace
- Discuss the impact that abusive behavior by and among healthcare professionals has on patient safety
- Describe the various studies related to behaviors that undermine a culture of safety
- Identify incidents of disrespectful communication or behavior and reframe them into respectful approaches
- Explain how communication strategies contribute to and alleviate emotional and physical abuse

- Lateral or horizontal violence
- Bullying
- Disruptive behavior
- Behaviors that undermine a culture of safety
- Toxic culture

Mutual respect among members of a healthcare workforce is integral to communicating effectively and in turn creating a healthy environment in which patient safety and patient experience are the top priorities. However, physical and emotional abuse in the workplace has been and continues to be a daunting problem in the world of healthcare, making many healthcare settings unsafe for patients and the people that provide care. Abusive or disrespectful behaviors among nurses, physicians, and other healthcare professionals are well documented. In addition, there are alarming statistics documenting occupational injuries to healthcare professionals at the hands of aggressive patients.

Not surprisingly, poor communication and/or deficits in emotional intelligence are factors in the predominance of abusive and disrespectful behavior. In this chapter, students will learn about the various types of inappropriate behavior, how such behaviors relate to communication, and what impact they have on the effort to provide safe, quality care. In addition, students will explore behaviors that undermine a culture of safety and develop skills in identifying, preventing, and addressing them.

TYPES OF ABUSIVE AND DISREPECTFUL BEHAVIOR

A physician belittles a nurse in front of a patient. A nurse manager tells the staff nurse she should not be so sensitive about a physician's angry outburst. A staff nurse avoids a conflict with a colleague but gossips about the situation with other colleagues. A unit coordinator rolls her eyes when the agency nurse asks a question about the overhead paging process. A scrub nurse decides not to mention a concern about the sponge count with the surgeon because he has a reputation for criticizing and making humiliating remarks. These are all occurrences of unprofessional and disrespectful communication. Sadly, such aggressive, passive-aggressive, and passive behaviors are commonplace in many organizations, and their presence compromises staff's ability to deliver safe, quality care. Beyond emotional abuse from colleagues, nurses are at risk for physical abuse from patients and their families as well, whether it is a husband who raises a threatening fist when demanding pain medicine for his wife or an out-of-control patient who physically strikes a nurse.

Any time there is a pervasive lack of open, honest, and respectful dialogue among professionals, there is likely to be suboptimal teamwork, more errors, and potential physical and psychological injuries to workers (discussed later in the chapter). Further, when healthcare professionals are seen being rude to each other, a message is given to all observers, including patients, that it is okay to treat others disrespectfully in healthcare settings.

There are many terms used in healthcare circles to describe various sources or types of abusive behavior: covert abuse, overt abuse, incivility, bad conduct, psychological violence, nonverbal or verbal abuse, and vertical abuse. Some of the more common terms are defined here; note how their definitions overlap and how all involve disrespectful verbal and/or nonverbal communication.

Lateral or Horizontal Violence

Lateral or horizontal violence is aggression (active or passive) among peers, such as a nurse bullying another nurse. It is not uncommon for nurses who may have been treated disrespectfully to take it out on more vulnerable peers such as recent grads, less confident colleagues, or nurses who are new to the team or organization. "Nurses eat their young" is a well-known phrase in the profession, referring to seasoned nurses who intimidate, discourage, or belittle newer nurses. The 10 most common forms of lateral violence in nursing are as follows:

- Nonverbal innuendo
- Verbal affront
- Undermining activities
- Withholding information
- Sabotage
- Infighting
- Scapegoating
- Backstabbing
- Failure to respect privacy
- Broken confidences (Griffin, 2004)

Estimates of lateral violence in the nursing workplace range from 46% to 100% (Stanley et al., 2007). Engaging in such behaviors may be easier and seem emotionally safer than risking a conflict, but it is not healthy for individuals, teams, and organizations providing care or for the patients receiving it.

Bullying

Bullying is classified as abusive behavior toward another that takes place repeatedly over time. Workplace bullying usually includes a real or perceived unequal power gradient, such as between a manager and staff nurse, among several staff members and a single staff member, and between a surgeon and an intern. This power can be abused in several ways: a surgeon who repeatedly berates members of the operating room team, a group of seasoned nurses that consistently excludes new staff from conversations, a nurse manager who shows favoritism to some staff and is overly critical of particular nurses, or a nurse who gives preferred treatment or assignments to assistants that she likes while disrespecting certain support staff.

Disruptive Behavior

Disruptive behavior is conduct by staff working in an organization that intimidates others to the extent that quality and safety could be compromised. In the *Case in Point Salary and Trends Special Report*, this author and Alan Rosenstein (2011) discuss the similarities and differences between nurse and physician disruptive behaviors. Although there are exceptions, nurses tend to be more passive-aggressive or passive, whereas physicians are more aggressive in their disruptive behaviors.

Behaviors That Undermine a Culture of Safety

In 2012, The Joint Commission stopped using the term *disruptive behavior* because of confusion and unfavorable opinions about the term, and replaced it with **behaviors that undermine a culture of safety**, which is considered any behavior that interferes with the open and honest exchange or seeking of information among healthcare staff and therefore poses a risk to safe, quality care. This includes withholding information, use of intimidating verbal and/or nonverbal language, talking about others behind their back, not listening to or considering constructive feedback, and tolerating such behaviors in others.

Consultant Commentary

Any time I facilitate discussions about workplace abuse among nurses in teaching or training situations, I hear stories about physicians throwing objects, yelling, or making inappropriate sexual advances; nurses gossiping, bullying, or "back-biting"; and patients screaming, pushing, punching, or worse. It seems as if all nurses have experienced some kind of abuse. Many years ago, I was a staff nurse caring for a physician who was recovering from surgery associated with advanced cancer and on a patient-controlled analgesia (PCA) pump with morphine. He was in a private room, and I went in to check his intravenous (IV) site. He was walking toward me, mumbling, and steadying himself with one hand on the IV pole. I backed away and found myself up against the wall as he reached out with both arms and put his hands around my neck. Being taller and steadier—while, at the same time, stunned—I took his hands, removed them from my neck, gently pushed him away, and got out of the room. The patient's surgeon (and also friend) was sitting at the nurses' station writing orders, and I told him what had happened. He told me his friend was having symptoms of withdrawal from the morphine, and he was changing the dose. So, what happened next? Nothing. At the time, I took the incident in stride and continued working. Only many years later, it occurred to me that the surgeon never asked me if I was okay, there was not any organizational effort to ensure my safety, and I wasn't offered support to address any emotional trauma that I may have experienced. Yet, I accepted it so readily as part of my job. Now I realize that even though there might have been reasons that this patient became abusive, it was not okay for him to treat me abusively.

Toxic Culture

Interrelated with workplace abuse is organizational culture (discussed in greater detail in Part III). Negative types of organizational cultures are **toxic cultures**, which can develop in a workplace where professional, paraprofessional, and support staff do not give and receive constructive feedback in a respectful way. In such a culture, bullying and blaming are unwritten rules of conduct, and a lack of mutual respect is rampant among individuals, teams, and departments. Communication skills are lacking, and abusive or disrespectful behavior is tolerated despite policies and signs that propose otherwise. Lack of awareness about and/or compassion for the impact behaviors have on others, beliefs and attitudes about superiority or inferiority, and unequal power dynamics or status differences permeate interactions in a negative way. Large egos boosted by power and status rather than expertise and leadership equate with being greater human beings. Weaker egos lacking in power and status resort to gossip, sabotage, and exclusion as a way to have a voice. Instead of collaboration, people form alliances, refuse to work with others, and build resentments, all of which take an emotional and physical toll.

STUDYING A PERVASIVE PROBLEM

Healthcare professionals practice, tolerate, excuse, avoid, and cope with disruptive behavior in many ways:

- "He was just venting after a very stressful day!"
- "I'm used to it. It helps to develop a thick skin."
- "She only threw the suture kit at him because he gave her the wrong one."
- "It's part of the job. That's what I tell the new grads."
- "I reported Dr. Smith's outburst to Human Resources twice last year, but no one ever did anything about it."
- "I don't have time to schedule a private conversation, and she won't listen anyway."
- "I'm going to wait and see if Mrs. Jones's blood pressure goes any lower. I really don't want to wake up the on-call doctor. He gets so angry."
- "His bedside manner is horrible, but he is a brilliant surgeon."

Healthcare staff at all levels may avoid being accountable for giving and receiving honest feedback, respecting difference, and learning from each other. It may feel less risky personally, and there may be an organizational pattern whereby it has been acceptable to blame others openly or behind their back rather than to show ownership and consider others' feelings in making decisions about behavior. Trust among staff in such environments is usually broken or precarious, and this presents serious limitations to interprofessional teamwork and patient outcomes. When conflicts are avoided rather than resolved, and when blaming others and avoiding responsibility become a priority over investigating underlying causes, nurses hesitate consciously or subconsciously to contact physicians at the first sign of trouble, and doctors get angry at nurses when they call *and* when they don't call. Whatever the case, patients miss out on getting the benefit of the entire healthcare team's expertise. Everyone suffers.

There are numerous studies that discuss the incidence, type, nomenclature, and source (i.e., physician or nurse) of disrespectful, abusive behavior in healthcare, and they also reveal its pervasiveness. One landmark survey was conducted by a regional office of VHA Inc., a national alliance of more than 1,400 not-for-profit hospitals. Unprecedented in size and scope, the survey, conducted from 2004 through 2007, included more than 4,500 participants across the

United States representing a variety of perspectives, including those of physicians, nurses, administrators, and other professionals from more than 102 hospitals. The survey focused directly on the impact that inappropriate behaviors have on psychological and behavioral reactions and how those may affect performance and consequently patient safety. The results were published in *The Joint Commission Journal on Quality and Patient Safety* (Rosenstein & O'Daniel, 2008) and included these statistics:

- 77% witnessed disruptive behavior from physicians (p. 465)
- 65% witnessed disruptive behavior from nurses (p. 465)
- 67% agreed that disruptive behaviors were linked to adverse events (p. 465)
- 71% agreed that disruptive behaviors were linked to medical errors (p. 466)
- 27% agreed that disruptive behaviors were linked to patient mortality (p. 466)

Interestingly, higher percentages of nurses witnessed disruptive behavior in physicians (88%) than witnessed disruptive behavior in nurses (73%) (p. 465). Possible reasoning for this difference is that disruptive behavior in nurses is less obvious.

Another large survey, conducted by the American College of Physician Executives and reported by Carrie Johnson (2009), involved 2,100 doctors and nurses. This study revealed similar links between behavior by professionals and the ability to collaborate for safe, quality patient care:

- Nearly 98% of the respondents witnessed behavior problems between doctors and nurses the previous year. (p. 6)
- About 30% said bad behavior occurred several times a year, 30% said it happened monthly, 25% said it happened weekly, and 10% said it happened every day. (p. 6)
- The percentages of respondents indicating specific types of behavior problems that they experienced at their healthcare organizations over the previous year were reported as follows (p. 8):
  - Degrading comments: 84.5%
  - Yelling: 73.0%
  - Cursing: 49.4%
  - Inappropriate joking: 45.5%
  - Refusing to work together: 38.4%
  - Refusing to speak to each other: 34.3%
  - Trying to get someone disciplined unjustly: 32.3%
  - Throwing objects: 18.9%
  - Trying to get someone fired unjustly: 18.6%
  - Spreading malicious rumors: 17.1%
  - Sexual harassment: 13.4%
  - Physical assault: 2.8%
  - Other: 10.0%

In July 2008, The Joint Commission (TJC) released a Sentinel Event Alert to address rising concerns regarding the incidence and impact of poor conduct among healthcare professionals (what was referred to in 2008 as *disruptive behavior* and in 2012 was revised to *behaviors that undermine a culture of safety* [TJC, 2012]). This was an exciting and formal step in raising awareness about the problem and creating a standard for good conduct. The alert connects inappropriate behaviors with poor patient outcomes, wasted costs, loss of qualified staff, and interference with the collaborative teamwork and culture needed to provide quality and safe care (TJC, 2008). The report cites multiple causes: a history of tolerance, indifference to the impact of disrespectful behaviors on others, productivity demands, power structures, fear of reporting, and professionals who have tendencies toward self-centeredness, immaturity, or defensiveness.

Most recently, the Lucian Leape Institute at the National Patient Safety Foundation released a roundtable report, *Through the Eyes of the Workforce: Creating Joy, Meaning, and Safer Health Care* (2013). The roundtable, consisting of more than 25 clinical and administrative leaders from all over the United States, took a serious look at the physical and psychological harm that the healthcare workforce is experiencing along with its connection to patient safety. What is unique about this report is its strong statement of advocacy for the workforce. Abusive behaviors undermine patient safety, but it is also important for nurses and other healthcare professionals to have rewarding *and* safe careers. Some of the most important findings are provided in the following excerpts taken from the executive summary of the report:

- "The prevalence of physical harm experienced by the healthcare workforce is striking, much higher than in other industries. Up to a third of nurses experience back or musculoskeletal injuries in a year, and many have unprotected contact with blood-borne pathogens." (p. ES1)

- "Psychological harm is also common. In many healthcare organizations, staff are not treated with respect—or worse yet, they are routinely treated with disrespect. Emotional abuse, bullying, and even threats of physical assault and learning by humiliation are all often accepted as 'normal' conditions of the healthcare workplace, creating a culture of fear and intimidation that saps joy and meaning from work." (p. ES1)

- "An environment of mutual respect is critical if the workforce is to find meaning and joy in work. In modern healthcare, teamwork is essential for safe practice, and teamwork is impossible in the absence of mutual respect." (p. ES2)

Confident Voices

Alan H. Rosenstein, MD, MBA
Healthcare Consultant

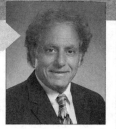

Improving Physician Communication Efficiency: Wants, Needs, and Strategies

Physicians, nurses, and staff are a precious resource, and we need to do what we can to continue to support them in what they want to do: gaining pride and respect for providing excellent patient care.

In the past, we have conducted extensive research on the adverse impact of physician disruptive behaviors on nurse relationships and clinical outcomes of care (Rosenstein & O'Daniel, 2005). Although progress has been made, there is still a long way to go. Beyond disruptive behaviors is the importance of improving overall

Continued

Confident Voices—cont'd

communication and collaboration efficiency. Policies, procedures, training, and intervention strategies help, but the real issue is to better understand the pressures influencing physician attitudes and behaviors that affect their role in providing patient care.

With growing complexities, technological advancements, specialized services, and cross-accountabilities for performance outcomes across the entire spectrum of care, the importance of effective communication and integrated team collaboration is more important than ever. Physicians play a pivotal role in this process. The need for connection and effective communication from physician to physician, physician to staff (nursing, case management, discharge planning, ancillary support services, and so on), and physician to patient and family is a crucial part of the treatment plan. The treatment plan needs to be consistent, consensus driven, and well organized in an effort to better coordinate care plans, set expectations, improve care efficiency and outcomes, improve overall satisfaction, and improve compliance with best practice care guidelines (Rosenstein, 2012a). Engaging, training, and involving physicians in this process are crucial for success. This sounds like the ideal thing to do, but unfortunately our experiences show that significant barriers still exist.

For physicians, there are several reasons that things are not going according to plan. Many of these start with medical training. Physicians gain confidence through dedicated study that emphasizes clinical knowledge expertise and technical competency. This leads to more autonomous, independent thinking and control and more autocratic and demanding types of behaviors, which are the antithesis of developing personal relationship skills to enhance communication and team collaboration experiences. One unwanted effect of this training is that physicians suffer from a lack of emotional intelligence, which perpetuates a unidirectional approach to care management that suffers from a lack of awareness and sensitivity of how they are affecting those they come into contact with. Fortunately, many medical schools are beginning to recognize the importance of developing personal relationship skills and are beginning to introduce training programs into the educational curriculum. Integrated healthcare networks, hospitals, and large medical groups should follow suit. Taking time to discuss with physicians the demands of today's healthcare environment, rallying around a positive culture with aligned objectives of patient-focused care, offering assistance and career support, providing training to enhance emotional intelligence, improving communication and collaboration skills, and offering other courses that may include diversity, stress, anger, or conflict management will go a long way in enhancing physician understanding and engagement.

One area of particular concern is the growing amount of stress and burnout accentuated by healthcare reform and other healthcare initiatives causing significant

Confident Voices—cont'd

changes in traditional models for care delivery. This may lead to ill effects on emotional and physical performance, which can affect motivation, satisfaction, efficiency, and work relationships and, in some cases, can even lead to negative impacts on patient care (Rosenstein, 2012b). Many physicians are frustrated, angry, and burned out to the point that they are losing interest, changing jobs, changing professions, or retiring prematurely. Organizations need to recognize the impact this is having on nurses and staff morale and take steps to provide assistance and support. One strategy is to set up a forum for discussion in which physicians can safely share their needs and concerns. In response, the organization can provide appropriate administrative, financial, or clinical support. For issues involving work–life balance, wellness, career objectives, and emotional or behavioral disturbances, the organization can provide support through a variety of coaching or counseling services programs offered through human resources, employee assistance programs, wellness committees, or outside resources that can effectively address issues related to stress, burnout, or other emotional or behavioral problems.

Given the growing pressures in today's environment, individuals, teams, and organizations need to take a proactive stance to help physicians, nurses, and all staff to find value and respect for what they do, restore their passions and energies for clinical care, improve satisfaction, improve work relationships, improve efficiency and productivity, and encourage wellness and work–life balance. Day-to-day efforts promoting the importance of efficient communication and respectful collaboration and its impact on patient care is essential for achieving these goals.

References

Rosenstein, A. H. (2012a). Physician communication and care management: The good, the bad, and the ugly. *Physician Executive Journal, 38*(4), 34–37.

Rosenstein, A. H. (2012b). Physician stress and burnout: What can we do? *American College of Physician Executives, 38*(6), 22–30.

Rosenstein, A. H., & O'Daniel, M. (2005). Disruptive behavior and clinical outcomes: Perceptions of nurses and physicians. *American Journal of Nursing, 105*(1), 54–64.

Biography

Dr. Alan Rosenstein, MD, MBA, is currently a practicing internist in San Francisco, medical director for physician wellness services in Minneapolis, and a consultant in healthcare management. Dr. Rosenstein has written more than 150 nationally recognized publications, and he has extensive national and international lecture and consultation experience in the areas of care management, clinical decision support, nurse–physician–staff relationships, communication efficiency, and behaviors affecting patient safety, quality, satisfaction, and clinical outcomes of care.

ABUSIVE AND DISRESPECTFUL BEHAVIOR FROM PATIENTS

Curbing workplace abuse among colleagues in a healthcare setting is not the only issue; controlling abuse of healthcare workers at the hands of patients is also critical. It is not uncommon for distraught family members or patients to engage in improper behavior toward nurses, such as yelling at a nurse, invading her personal space, or even physically assaulting her. Because of dependency and vulnerability issues (discussed in Chapter 6), patients and families may be overwhelmed with stress. Hours of waiting met by a nurse who is in a hurry may fuel heightened emotional states that trigger an inappropriate response by patients or their families. Patients with dementia and mental health problems and those who may be intoxicated or suffering from metabolic disorders may be especially challenging.

Although the fears and anxieties of patients are completely understandable, expressions of anger and violence are not appropriate and make the practice of nursing risky at times. Further, when nurses spend time and energy dealing with aggressive patients, it also takes them away from other patients and creates stress, which is likely to affect quality patient care. Abuse against a nurse by a patient also demonstrates poor behavior to others and, when not challenged, implies such behavior is acceptable. Anyone who has ever worked in an in-patient group setting, such as a dementia unit, can attest to the contagious influence that aggressive behaviors can have on a community. One person acting up is unsettling and contributes to anxiety and agitation in others. Passive or passive-aggressive behaviors can also be contagious because they, too, set a precedent for how people behave and communicate.

Most concerning is physical assault by patients and their families, and these statistics reveal how serious the problem is:

- A nurse or doctor has a five to six times higher chance of being assaulted than a cab driver in an urban area (Lucian Leape Institute, 2013, p. 10).

- In a 2011 health and safety survey of more than 4,600 nurses, 11% of respondents reported having been physically assaulted in the previous 12 months, whereas just over 50% said they had been threatened or verbally abused. Additionally, about one-third of those surveyed listed on-the-job assault as one of their top three safety concerns. All of these statistics showed increased percentages compared with results from a 2001 survey (American Nurses Association [ANA], 2011).

As awareness and concern are growing about this problem, many states are considering or enacting legislation designed to address it, such as mandating prevention programs, making it a felony to assault a healthcare worker, and increasing fines for doing so (Rice, 2014). The ANA (2014) has compiled a list of states engaged in legislative action to investigate workplace violence against healthcare workers.

Healthcare administration must do its part as well to address the problem. Staffing ratios that allow for timely attention to patient needs, proactive communication of updates regarding patient status, and listening respectfully to staff and patient concerns will help minimize anxiety and prevent escalating panic and aggression. A nurse liaison available to keep family informed during an emergency or clinical crisis is a staffing measure that demonstrates organizational concern for workforce safety and health as well as a high standard of care for patients. An armed security guard in an emergency department sends a powerful nonverbal message to all that inappropriate behavior will not be tolerated. However, such staffing represents a challenge for leaders trying to make cost-effective decisions about paying for staff that may only be needed some of the time.

In addition, giving clear messages by role-modeling respectful interprofessional behavior and, when necessary, disciplining offenders will help to dispel the myth that it is okay to be abusive to healthcare personnel.

CHANGING ABUSIVE BEHAVIOR USING RESPECTFUL COMMUNICATION

Whether physical or emotional, whether at the hands of a colleague or a patient, abusive and disrespectful behavior and its damaging consequences to the healthcare workforce and patients are begging for solutions that address the underlying problems. A behavioral approach to communication is a fundamental part of the answer. The following scenarios portray the use of respectful communication skills and professional behaviors in response to disrespectful behavior among nurses and physicians.

Being Assertive and Listening Respectfully

A physician runs into a nurse on her way to a code and tells her to "Get the hell out of the way." The nurse obliges but seeks out the physician the next day and has the following exchange:

"Doctor, I'd like to talk with you briefly about our run-in yesterday when you were en route to a code. Do you have a few minutes sometime today?"

"I can talk with you now. What's up?"

"I was frustrated with the way you pushed me aside and told me to 'Get the hell out of the way.' I understand that you were in a rush, but I deserve to be treated respectfully."

"I guess that was pretty rude. Sorry."

In this instance, the nurse is being assertive, and the physician is listening respectfully. The whole dialogue takes very little time, with the result being that they walk away respecting each other. An ideal solution, this mutually respectful and brief conversation between the parties involved nips the problem in the bud and allows the relationship between nurse and physician to develop in a positive way. The situation could have followed other less ideal paths, of course. If the nurse had not spoken up, the physician may have never realized how her behavior was perceived. Meanwhile, the nurse would have probably held onto some feelings of being mistreated and may have talked about the doctor with colleagues. Similar situations may have recurred and a dysfunctional pattern perpetuated. If the physician had refused to have a conversation or had been defensive, the nurse could have discussed the issue with the unit manager. Provided that the nurse manager has the skill set and is supported by senior leaders for addressing concerns about conduct, a facilitated meeting with the staff nurse and physician could be held. Eventually representatives from human resources and/or the union would need to get involved, depending on protocols for grievance processes.

Giving and Receiving Feedback

In a related scenario, a staff nurse feeling frustrated with a physician's angry outburst brings her concerns to the nurse manager. The nurse manager comments, "It sounds like the doctor's behavior is bothering you a lot. I can understand your feeling angry and hurt. I'd like to work with you as a coach and help you prepare some feedback to provide him. It will be a hard but important conversation." The nurse manager has validated the staff nurse and, at the same time, engages her in a plan to address her concerns and build a positive relationship with the physician. Knowing she has the support of senior leaders, the nurse feels supported in calling the physician on his behavior, leading to meaningful learning for both parties when she confronts him, as shown in the following dialogue:

"Doctor, I'd like to talk with you in the next day or two about our phone conversation regarding our patient yesterday. When would you have a few minutes?"

"I have about 3 minutes right now. Can we be quick?"

"Yes. I called you during office hours about the patient because I was concerned about her increase in blood pressure and history of CVA. I felt your tone was abrupt and that you were dismissive of my concerns. I want to feel comfortable calling you with concerns about our patients. What are your thoughts?"

"I remember you calling and feeling frustrated with our conversation, too. I was in the middle of three urgent issues and that patient's blood pressure was only slightly elevated. I want you to feel comfortable calling me, too, but that call felt unnecessary."

"I'd be happy to honor any parameters and would appreciate it if you would treat me and my concerns with respect. Does that sound reasonable? What parameters would you advise?"

"I understand and will work to convey respect when you call. Call if her systolic is greater than 160 or diastolic is greater than 90."

"I'll record your orders in the computer so that everyone will be clear."

"Thank you."

This exchange included the giving and receiving of feedback, which offers all sorts of learning opportunities. The physician is given feedback that he can keep in mind for future conversations with nurses. Meanwhile, the nurse learns or is reminded to clarify parameters with this doctor and others as well as how to better develop judgment about contacting physicians. If the physician's behavior continues over time, the nurse and the nurse manager can consider more formal procedures, as mentioned in the previous scenario.

Defusing a Physical Threat

A less common scenario is a nurse facing a physical threat. When faced with a physical threat, getting out of danger is always the priority, and calling security or running away certainly trump communication strategies in those circumstances. But to prevent such situations in the first place or to defuse expressions of anger before they escalate to physical violence, respectful communication is vital. Although stand-alone workshops and psychiatric nursing courses cover this topic more completely, a brief discussion is warranted here.

Nurses must learn to recognize the signs of anger, such as a sudden change in affect, reddening face, invasion of another's personal space, and clenching fists. If these emotional cues are identified early enough, it is possible to address them and prevent further escalation with a simple validation: "I know you have been waiting a long time. It looks like you're getting angry." Respectful listening may be all it takes to defuse a patient's intense emotions, especially when followed by an offer to move things along or an explanation for the wait. Also, using nonthreatening body language and a confident but gentle tone can portray a willingness to listen without suggesting vulnerability. (Portraying a lack of confidence may inadvertently give permission for escalating expressions of anger.)

On the other hand, demonstrating authority is sometimes very effective in containing aggression. Provided physical safety is less of a concern, as with a security guard located in a nearby room, a nurse can address an act of aggression by stating, "Stop!" using a firm voice, a confident stance, and a strong gesture, such as putting an arm out with palm facing the aggressor.

Regardless of the scenario, a strong focus on respectful communication is key to eliminating bullying, minimizing violence, and building safe cultures. However, it is important to keep in mind that what is effective in one situation may be less so in another, and this mainly depends on the people and circumstances involved. Further, what works in one relationship may fail in another. Differences or commonalities between individuals, such as personality, height, age, or ethnicity, can all come into play. Human dynamics are very complicated, so nurses will have to use at least some level of intuition. The more nurses can recognize emotional cues from others and remain sensitive as to how their behaviors affect others, the more effectively they will be able to use communication to deflate escalating situations.

CASE STUDY

Sarah is an RN caring for a patient who has just had a total abdominal hysterectomy and is recovering on the medical-surgical floor. On the patient's second postoperative day, Sarah is distracted and picks up a soiled wound gauze from the floor after discarding her gloves. Unknown to Sarah, the patient witnesses the act and complains to the surgeon, who tells her such behavior is unacceptable and that he will find out who is to blame for this incompetence. The surgeon then proceeds to berate the nurse manager: "Your nursing staff is incompetent and unprofessional, and I want the person responsible off this unit." The nurse manager finds Sarah later that day and reprimands her: "How will we ever stop these complaints when you do something as stupid as that?" Sarah is very upset and unfocused when she enters the same patient's room to give her an intramuscular injection, which makes the patient, in turn, even more anxious. After her discharge, the patient completes a hospital survey and gives the unit a poor score. A few weeks later, the chief executive officer of the hospital is reviewing survey feedback and notes a poor score on this unit. She holds a meeting with the chief nursing officer and the nurse manager to investigate. The nurse manager recalls the incident involving Sarah. All agree that Sarah must be disciplined.

Discussion Questions

1. List any opportunities that the healthcare professionals in this case study missed for giving and receiving direct feedback. How might the outcome have been different in each instance?

2. Do you believe a patient should give constructive feedback to a nurse? Support your reasoning.

3. How would you describe the relationships of the people involved in the case study?

SUMMARY

A demoralizing and insidious part of the healthcare culture, abusive and disrespectful behavior has a destructive influence on relationships, communication, and safety. Incidences of inappropriate behavior that take place in healthcare settings demonstrate a lack respect for self and for others. Being aware of how behaviors are perceived is a valuable skill. Training, practice, and enforcement of respectful communication to include a focus on giving and receiving constructive feedback will go a long way toward eliminating or at least minimizing inappropriate behaviors among professionals and patients and their families. As awareness about inappropriate behavior and how effective communication skills can stop such incidences increases among all healthcare professionals, there will be fewer toxic cultures. When healthcare professionals and organizations master effective communication strategies and when respectful communication behaviors are the norm, it will be easier to set clear expectations for behavior from patients, families, and visitors.

Reflection Questions

1. Have you ever observed behavior by a healthcare professional that undermined a culture of safety? How could communication have been used to diffuse the situation?

2. Have you ever lost your temper or patience with a classmate or colleague? What were the circumstances surrounding the issue? How do you think it might have affected the other person and any witnesses? What might you do differently after reading this chapter? Why?

3. Consider the questions above as if *you* are the one who has been treated disrespectfully or witnessed a colleague or classmate who has been.

References

American Nurses Association. (2011). 2011 ANA health and safety survey. *Nursing World.* Retrieved from www.nursingworld.org/MainMenuCategories/WorkplaceSafety/Healthy-Work-Environment/SafeNeedles/2011-HealthSafetySurvey.html

American Nurses Association. (2014). Workplace violence. Retrieved from www.nursingworld.org/workplaceviolence.

Boynton, B., & Rosenstein, A. H. (2011). Disruptive behavior: Differences between physicians and nurses—what case managers should know. *Case in Point Salary and Trends Special Report.*

Griffin, M. (2004). Teaching cognitive rehearsal as a shield for lateral violence: An intervention for newly licensed nurses. *Journal of Continuing Education in Nursing, 35*(6), 257–263.

Johnson, C. (2009). Bad blood: Doctor-nurse behavior problems impact patient care. *Physician Executive Journal, 35*(6), 6–11. Retrieved from www.ache.org/policy/doctornursebehavior.pdf

The Joint Commission. (2008). Behaviors that undermine a culture of safety. *Sentinel Event Alert, 40.* Retrieved from www.jointcommission.org/sentinel_event_alert_issue_40_behaviors_that_undermine_a_culture_of_safety

The Joint Commission. (2012). Leadership standard clarified to address behaviors that undermine a safety culture. *The Joint Commission Perspectives, 32*(1), 7.

Lucian Leape Institute. (2013). *Through the eyes of the workforce: Creating joy, meaning, and safer health care.* Boston: National Patient Safety Foundation. Retrieved from www.npsf.org/wp-content/uploads/2013/03/Through-Eyes-of-the-Workforce_online.pdf

National Center on Elder Abuse. (n.d.) Retrieved from www.ncea.aoa.gov

Rice, S. (2014, February 14). States increasingly trying to protect healthcare workers from violence. *Modern Healthcare.* Retrieved from www.modernhealthcare.com/article/20140214/NEWS/302149971

Rosenstein, A. H., & O'Daniel, M. (2008). A survey of the impact of disruptive behaviors and communication defects on patient safety. *The Joint Commission Journal on Quality and Patient Safety, 34*(8), 464–471.

Stanley K. M., Martin M. M., Nemeth, L. S., Michel, Y., & Welton, M. (2007). Examining lateral violence in the nursing workplace. *Issues in Mental Health Nursing, 28*(11), 1247–1265.

CHAPTER 8

Managing Stress and Strategies for Self-Care

LEARNING OUTCOMES

- Recognize the importance of self-care among nurses
- Describe the physical, psychological, and cognitive demands of nursing and identify ways to manage stress around them
- Explain how emotional intelligence and effective communication can make stress motivating and decrease harmful stress
- Discuss the importance of standardized communication during stressful and emergency situations

KEY TERMS

- Self-care
- Burnout
- Compassion fatigue
- Caregiving
- Caretaking
- Codependence
- Cognitive stacking

Nursing is a high-stakes, high-stress, and yet rewarding profession with intense cognitive, physical, and emotional demands. State-of-the-art technology, cutting-edge procedures, adventurous specialties with travel opportunities, and the privilege of providing distinguished service are all part of this dynamic career. There are also pervasive stressors associated with professional nursing: exposure to tragedy and loss, relentlessly urgent action, constant change, information overload, and overwhelming workloads. All of these stimulating, rewarding demands can easily turn into unhealthy and even debilitating stress. For nurses to consistently provide a high standard of patient-centered care and sustain long-lasting, rewarding careers, it is necessary to be familiar with common stressors of nursing practice and know how to manage them, remember the importance of health and well-being, and practice self-care strategies. This chapter will explore the importance of effective communication in dealing with common stressors in nursing and examine the underlying emotional intelligence necessary for managing stress and maintaining a healthy work–life balance.

SELF-CARE

Optimal health and well-being should be a priority for student and practicing nurses. After all, promoting health is the business nurses are in. The only way to achieve this is through **self-care**. Physical and psychological health require adequate rest, exercise, good nutrition, positive relationships, stress management, an ability to reflect and learn, and time for fun. Nurses who come to work rested, fit, and emotionally secure are poised to provide safe and compassionate care. In addition, they model important lifestyle behaviors for colleagues and patients, are less susceptible to damage caused by psychological and physical workplace harms, and are overall happier. Self-care arises out of emotional intelligence and assertiveness. An awareness of what one needs, a sense of self-worth, and an ability to ask for support are all important to safe care, optimal patient experience, and long-term, rewarding careers. That is not to say that anyone with less than perfect health habits or emotional intelligence should be judged or reprimanded. In fact, self-acceptance and acceptance of others are foundational to positive health behavioral changes for nurses and the patients they work with.

Self-care helps nurses to value their own health as well as that of patients, friends, and families—an investment that involves spending time, money, and emotional energy. The American Holistic Nurses Association (2014) is a proponent of self-care, which it believes can be achieved through the following:

- Body: Exercise, grooming, massages, breathing, yoga, conscious eating
- Mind: Quiet contemplation, meditation, focusing on the moment, healing music, laughter
- Spirit: Meditation and prayer, reading spiritual literature, listing positive things in your life, random acts of kindness

A wide variety of physical, emotional, and spiritual resources await nurses seeking to inspire, improve, or continue self-care. Over the last several years, more nurses have started businesses in the health and wellness arena. There are nurses who offer nutritional counseling, teach mediation and yoga, and more. Some have become nurse coaches or nurse psychotherapists and help craft and encourage self-care strategies or address issues related to burnout. Employer wellness programs, employee health nurses, and employee assistance programs are all potential resources that may be available in healthcare facilities. There may be similar tools available to nursing students in their programs.

Confident Voices

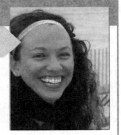

Elizabeth Scala, MSN, MBA, RN
Owner, Nursing from Within

Nursing From Within: Your Inner Guidance System to Whole-Person Self-Care

When I was asked to write about self-care for nurses and why it is important that we make ourselves a priority, two immediate thoughts came to mind:

1. What do I write? As nurses we *know* the information. We teach it to our patients and clients all day long. We know what "healthy" is and what it is not.

Confident Voices—cont'd

2. Yikes! That is a very broad topic with a vast amount of possibility. How do I approach this in a way that captures everything that we as nurses need to know?

I have decided to tackle this topic in a way that not only illustrates the whole-person perspective but also gives a broad overview of how the Nursing From Within model creates healthy living for us all. (If you are interested, you can find out more about the Nursing From Within model by visiting elizabethscala.com). To do this, let us discuss what self-care is and why it is so important.

What?

Often when we hear the term *self-care*, our minds immediately perceive physical things such as healthy eating or physical exercise. And although as nurses we know that this is important, I want to stress that these components are not the only things that make us truly happy and healthy nurses.

In addition, this narrow perspective can be the very thing that keeps us from enjoying healthy behaviors in the first place. For example, if you are a person who does not enjoy exercise or really hates to cook, then how are you going to partake in self-care if all you have is this narrow view of the physical realm?

Let me encourage you to think about what "healthy" is for you. Does it mean spending time outside in nature? Listening to relaxing music while taking a bubble bath? Self-care can be approached from a highly holistic perspective, from which we can enjoy making ourselves a priority in the physical, mental, emotional, spiritual, and energetic realms.

Why?

Why is a very important aspect of the self-care discussion—maybe even the most crucial component. The "why" behind what we do can be the make-or-break factor. It makes us reflect on our own motivation, or lack thereof: Why am I always putting other people before me? Why have I let my physical health go? What is going to make me motivated to make healthier choices for myself?

In addition to taking the time for introspection, we can also apply the concepts of the Nursing From Within model to this dialogue. When I created the Nursing From Within model, I was looking for a process that nurses could relate to. Nursing From Within truly applies taking care of and getting to know oneself in order to allow this love and light to ripple out to the world.

Nursing From Within involves mindset shifts and the opening of the heart in order to invite peace, joy, and balance in one's life. When we take care of ourselves from the inside out, we are truly empowered helpers and healers for all of those we come

Continued

Confident Voices—cont'd

in contact with. When we realize our own inner motivations for taking care of self, we can best take care of others.

Nursing is an amazing profession, one that I am entirely honored and completely proud to be a part of. We touch the lives of so many—often more than we ever can imagine or will ever know.

Our own self-care is so important; in fact, one could argue it is critical, because we are the face of healthcare. As nurses, we are with our patients around-the-clock. We are the eyes and ears of the system. We are patient advocates, patient teachers, and mindful listeners.

It is imperative that we take care of ourselves so that we can role-model what this looks and feels like to the public as a whole. It is our duty as nurse professionals to take care of ourselves so that we can best serve the world we live in.

Biography

Spiritual Practice Nurse Elizabeth Scala, MSN/MBA, RN, is on a mission to shift the profession of nursing from the inside out. As a speaker, author, workshop facilitator, and retreat leader, Scala inspires nursing teams to reconnect with the passionate and fulfilling joy that once called them to their roles. She is also a Reiki Master Teacher, certified coach, and the host of the virtual nursing conference called the Art of Nursing. When not speaking to or teaching other nurses, you can find her enjoying nature, practicing yoga, or dancing to her favorite jam band, moe. She can be reached via coachscala@livingsublimewellness.com

THE DEMANDS OF NURSING AND STRESS

Self-care is absolutely critical in battling the most common job hazard for nurses: stress. In 2011, more than 4,500 nurses responded to a survey conducted by the American Nurses Association (ANA) regarding the health and safety of nurses. The resulting report, outlined in the *American Nurse Today* (ANA, 2012), revealed that the top concern regarding workplace health and safety was the "effects of stress and overwork" (para. 3). In a similar survey 10 years earlier, also by the ANA (2001), the top safety concern of more than 4,800 respondents was the "acute/chronic effects of stress and overwork" (p. 3).

Stress in the day-to-day practice of nursing is nothing new. To some extent, this is the nature of the nurse professional's work. Part of every nurse's commitment to the profession includes awareness and acceptance of this reality. However, managing stress is critical because relentless stress without healthy coping strategies and rejuvenation can take a huge toll on a nurse's physical and psychological health. It can drain the joy and meaning out of providing care and negatively influence the nurse's ability to do so safely.

The National Institute for Occupational Safety and Health (1999) defines job stress as "the harmful physical and emotional responses that occur when the requirements of the job do not match the capabilities, resources, or needs of the worker" (para. 6). Nurses who do not manage ongoing job stress are more likely to eat poorly, smoke cigarettes, and abuse drugs or alcohol (Burke, 2000). These unhealthy coping mechanisms, along with the physical and psychological harms of excessive stress, contribute to a very long list of individual and work-place problems. Well documented in the literature, job stress includes negative interrelated consequences for nurses, patients, and organizations, such as absenteeism, poor concentration, costly staff turnover, medication errors, horizontal violence, and difficulty sleeping, just to name a few.

To practice self-care, nurses must first recognize the many physical, psychological, and cognitive demands of their job and then learn how to combat related stresses and/or stressors.

Physical Demands

From a physical standpoint, patient care is extremely demanding on nurses. The report, *Through the Eyes of the Workforce: Creating Joy, Meaning, and Safer Health Care,* from the Lucian Leape Institute at National Patient Safety Foundation (2013), indicates that "the prevalence of physical harm experienced by the healthcare workforce is striking, much higher than in other industries" (p. ES1). During a standard shift, nurses are often required to do heavy lifting and to bend, stoop, walk, and stand for prolonged hours. Significant manual dexterity is also required for measuring medication, starting intravenous lines, inserting catheters, and numerous other tasks. The presence of equipment, patients' personal belongings, and concerned family and friends make patients' rooms tight quarters. At night, many nurses work in poor light rather than risk waking up a sleep-deprived patient.

Assertive communication is an essential way for nurses to minimize risk for injury and optimize physical health. Nurses must ask for, offer, and accept help in physically taxing or unsafe situations, and they should even refuse to do something if help is not available.

Confident Voices

Dev Raheja, MS, CSP
President/Consultant of Patient System Safety

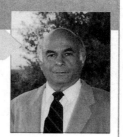

Safety of Nurses Improves Patient Safety and Quality

Nursing ranks among the worst occupations in terms of work-related injuries, and studies have shown that in a given year, nearly half of all nurses will have struggled with lower back pain. When nurses suffer, so do their patients. The cost to hospitals is enormous. Extrapolating the individual costs of these lapses in care to a national level, re-searchers estimate that medication errors and patient falls that occurred as a result of nurses' health issues incurred as much as $2 billion annually on the healthcare system: "We have money bleeding out the back door because we don't have a healthy work force," said Susan Letvak, an associate professor of nursing at the University of North Carolina at Greensboro (Chen, 2012, para. 14).

Many nurses may not want to admit it, but pain contributes to fatigue and can be distracting when caring for a patient. Combined with other fatigue such as work-ing long hours, psychological harm from doctors, and hearing what seems like a

Continued

Confident Voices—cont'd

1,000 alarms a day (of which more than 90% are not urgent), a nurse will be emotionally injured when he or she cannot respond to a patient in a crisis situation. Fatigue contributed to more than 1,600 events reported to Pennsylvania Patient Safety Authority alone since 2004; 37 of those incidents were adverse events, with 4 of them leading to patient deaths. Medication errors and mistakes related to a procedure, treatment, or test made up 88.5% of the events related to fatigue. The most significant error risk involves nurses working 12.5 hours or longer (MacDonald, 2014). Note that these are just the reported errors. Unreported errors are 10 times higher.

The Joint Commission (2011), through a Sentinel Event Alert, reports that fatigued workers can exhibit the following conditions:

- Lapses in attention and inability to stay focused
- Reduced motivation
- Compromised problem-solving
- Confusion
- Irritability
- Memory lapses
- Impaired communication
- Slowed or faulty information processing and judgment
- Diminished reaction time
- Indifference and loss of empathy

So what can be done proactively? Following are some suggestions that should improve the quality of care and safety of patients.

The primary efforts to implement regulations and guidelines to address healthcare worker fatigue has targeted limiting hours worked, but a more comprehensive approach is needed. Growing awareness of the risks for fatigue in the nursing industry has led The Joint Commission to issue a directive to all healthcare organizations to undertake a fatigue risk assessment and implement a fatigue risk management plan (Circadian 24/7 Work Force Solutions, 2014).

Nurse infections are also an important issue. They are exposed to methicillin-resistant *Staphylococcus aureus* (MRSA) and *Clostridium difficile* infections. They should be encouraged to get a swab test annually. Hospitals should sanitize surfaces like door knobs, toilet handles, bed rails, call buttons, and so on with the proper sanitizers. For example, *C. difficile* bacteria have to be eliminated through bleach-based sanitizers only; just alcohol will not do (Pomerance Berl, 2013).

Depression is a significant issue. One in eight U.S. workers has been diagnosed with depression, according to a recent Gallup poll. Many of them "look perfectly fine

Confident Voices—cont'd

yet are suffering tremendously on the inside," said David Mischoulon, a staff psychiatrist at Massachusetts General Hospital and Harvard Medical School. Under the Americans With Disabilities Act of 1990, employers must make reasonable accommodations for an employee suffering from major depression. The U.S. Centers for Disease Control and Prevention recommend that employers implement health-related services for depression. These include employee assistance programs that offer counseling to workers with depression and training to help managers better recognize the signs and symptoms (Gupta, 2014).

The best thing hospitals can do is engage nurses in incidence reporting. Any time that physical or psychological harm is experienced, it should be reported with suggestions for preventing such harm. If a hospital does not have such a system, nurses should speak up at an opportune time to those with authority. The only way to ensure the best patient-centered care is to have nurses who are healthy and, therefore, experience joy in their work.

References

Chen, P. W. (2012, July 5). When it's the nurse who needs looking after. *New York Times*. Retrieved from well.blogs.nytimes.com/2012/07/05/when-its-the-nurse-who-needs-looking-after/?_php=true&_type=blogs&_r=0

Circadian 24/7 Work Force Solutions. (2014). *Nursing and health care: Managing fatigue*. Retrieved from www.circadian.com/247-industries/health-care.html.

Gupta, S. (2014, January 9). Depression in the workplace: How companies and employees can address the condition's toll on mental health and productivity. *Everyday Health*. Retrieved from tinyurl.com/qd6psqe.

The Joint Commission. (2011, December 14). *Sentinel event alert issue 48: Health care worker fatigue and patient.* Retrieved from http://www.jointcommission.org/sea_issue_48/

MacDonald, I. (2014, July 5). Healthcare worker fatigue contributes to 1,600 patient safety events in Pennsylvania. *FierceHealthcare.* Retrieved from www.fiercehealthcare.com/story/healthcare-worker-fatigue-contributes-1600-patient-safety-events-pennsylvan/2014-06-05.

Pomerance Berl, R. (2013, March 25). How to keep your loved one safe in the hospital. *U. S. News and World Report*. Retrieved from health.usnews.com/health-news/health-wellness/articles/2013/03/25/how-to-keep-your-loved-one-safe-in-the-hospital

Biography

Dev Raheja, MS, CSP, has been a System Safety and System Reliability Engineering consultant for more than 25 years. His range of consulting encompasses transportation

Continued

Confident Voices—cont'd

systems, medical systems, and consumer products. He is the author of several books, including *Safer Hospital Care: Strategies for Continuous Innovation* (2011, Productivity Press); *Assurance Technologies Principles and Practices*, 2nd edition (2006, Wiley); and *Design for Reliability* (2012, Wiley). A Fellow of the System Safety Society, he has received a Scientific Achievement Award and the Educator-of the-Year Award from the society.

Psychological Demands

Emotionally, psychologically, and spiritually, nurses are in privileged places with patients. Although they often experience the fulfilling rewards of helping patients recover and cope, they also must endure the disappointments when unable to alleviate patient suffering or prevent loss. Burnout and compassion fatigue are examples of job-related psychological stresses that nurses may experience.

Burnout is described as emotional exhaustion, depersonalization, and reduced personal accomplishment (Maslach & Jackson, 1996). It involves an organizational component in that it is often a cumulative response to working in a chronically understaffed situation in which, no matter how hard the nurses try, they may not be able to complete all assignments in a way they find satisfactory. While wearily driving home from work, many nurses have experienced heart-sinking feelings when remembering a medication that was forgotten or a patient's report of pain that was not passed along to the next shift. If this is once in a while, a nurse learns from it and moves on. But if this happen every day, a nurse's ability to recover may diminish over time and a feeling of helplessness may settle in, which is not good for the nurse or her patients.

Compassion fatigue is a form of burnout associated with the relationships that nurses have with patients and families. These relationships can drain nurses physically, emotionally, and spiritually. Without good psychological boundaries, the empathy nurses have for patients can become a double-edged sword. Some nurses become so empathetic that they begin to actually feel the pain, loss, or suffering that patients and families experience.

Burnout, including compassion fatigue, can manifest in a variety of ways and affect the individual as well as teams and organizations. Symptoms include exhaustion, sadness, hopelessness, cynicism, boredom, irritability, desensitization, proneness to injuries, somatic complaints, poor performance, absenteeism, weight loss or gain, substance abuse, and other signs and symptoms of distress (Boyle, 2011).

Most commonly, burnout occurs when the line between caregiving and caretaking is crossed. **Caregiving** is the actual work nurses do, for which they receive pay, benefits, and other rewards in exchange for their time and expertise as well as joy and satisfaction from helping others. **Caretaking** arises when helping others is a compulsion that is consciously or subconsciously connected to meeting one's own needs, such as self-esteem, a sense of belonging, or a need to be loved. Although these needs can be met as a consequence of providing care, it is not healthy to seek, expect, require, or depend on it. Caretaking often involves a lack of self-care or excessive self-sacrifice, and the nursing profession offers almost constant exposure to patients who have multiple, possibly endless needs with limited resources. Therefore, in the case of caretaking, nurses develop a codependent relationship with their patients.

In the book, *I'm Dying to Take Care of You: Nurses and Codependence—Breaking the Cycles*, Candace Snow and David Willard (1989) offer a detailed description of **codependence**, self-assessment tools, and an action plan for addressing personal and organizational codependence. In the more recent article, "When Caregiving Ignites Burnout: New Ways to Douse the Flames," Rick Gessler and Liz Ferron (2012) discuss codependency in nursing and its contribution to burnout, bullying, and diminished morale among the healthcare team. The article makes the case for "unprecedented levels of job stress" (para. 2) in today's nurse practice settings and provides further discussion of problems associated with unhealthy degrees of self-sacrifice.

Developing self-awareness and respect for your feelings is integral to developing your emotional intelligence. Knowing what excess stress feels like, and that it is perfectly fine to feel it and to ask for help or a break in a respectful manner, combines emotional intelligence with assertiveness. This is likely to be easier for some than others. Spending time reflecting, journaling about experiences that involve stress and feelings, or sharing challenges with a friend or colleague may be sufficient ways of developing self-awareness and self-worth. For others, it helps to have a personal or professional coach who will help identify related strengths and opportunities for growth while supporting the development of assertiveness. Some individuals may find psychotherapy helpful to uncover and cope with underlying experiences that may contribute to false messages about inadequacy or lack of self-worth and to help develop a sense of self, one that is worthy of setting limits, asking for help, and maintaining personal boundaries.

Cognitive Demands

The cognitive demands of nursing involve the organizing, prioritizing, and decision-making involved in patient care, including but not limited to clinical information, workflow, nursing interventions and assessments, time management, productivity expectations, familiarity with patients and families, teamwork, troubleshooting equipment, and finding supplies. These tasks must be completed under varying amounts of uncertainty, frequent interruptions, and constantly shifting priorities, all of which fall under the term **cognitive stacking**. According to nurse researcher Patricia Ebright (2010), "[cognitive] stacking is the invisible, decision-making work of RNs about the what, how, and when of delivering nursing care to an assigned group of patients" (para. 9). Figuring out how to make a plan, execute it, and adapt it to new priorities is something that's going on in nurses' minds all the time.

Ebright explains that failure to understand the dynamic and complex process of cognitive stacking will lead to processes, environments, and technologies that complicate rather than support RN work. This in turn will contribute to "increased RN stress and dissatisfaction, decreased RN retention, and ultimately unsafe care" (para. 2).

One way for students to understand cognitive stacking is to think about, or better yet ask practicing nurses, what is going on in their mind as they plan their day and how they shift priorities in response to events. As the seasoned nurse plans a shift, some of this invisible thinking, organizing, and prioritizing include the following:

- Who are my patients, and what special circumstances should I be attentive to, such as a visit from hospice or physical therapy?
- When are their medications due? What are the treatments they need? Can I consolidate these tasks?
- What labs do I need to follow up on?
- Are there particular physicians whom I need to speak with and particular times they might be available?

- Will I need help or equipment for any tasks? Who is working today that I can ask for help? Can I save a few steps by getting supplies for one patient en route to visiting another?
- What might be a good learning experience for a student nurse who is following me?
- What can I delegate to the nurse assistant?

All of these are subject to change because of a new admission, a nurse who goes home sick, or a shift in one patient's clinical status. In addition, many have relationship components, such as positive or negative histories with physicians, colleagues, or assistants. The ability for RNs to stack effectively requires sophisticated clinical knowledge and judgment and a constant awareness of changes in patients and the environment, also known as *situational awareness*. Making the decision to postpone a dressing change and insulin injection for two patients because one patient is showing subtle signs warranting closer observation is a complex one. The nurse must consider potential ramifications of the tasks not done for all three patients and reprioritize, delegate, or ask for help. Delegation may depend on staffing in terms of both the numbers of nurses available and relationship histories. Influencing factors for a nurse considering asking for help would include, but not be limited to, feelings of alienation arising in part from gossip and feelings of inadequacy arising in part from constructive feedback received from a manager about time management.

Cognitive stacking includes ensuring safe and quality care as well as completing tasks and documentation on time. As if cognitive stacking weren't stressful enough on its own, additional stress may arise from an endless stream of challenges, such as new information regarding computer systems, emergent changes in patients' conditions, confusing physician orders, an emotionally intense conflict with family or colleagues, unfamiliarity with a treatment or procedure, and policy changes, among others. These in turn are influenced by human factors such as hunger, fatigue, anxiety, pain, and motivation.

Confidence, mindfulness, experience, knowledge, and clinical reasoning are tools nurses must use to counteract the ongoing stress of cognitive stacking. Although organizations can do more to optimize the environment in which nurses work in and, as will be explored in later chapters, address issues such as adequate staffing, safety engineering of the workplace, workflow design, and continuing education, nurses must use emotional intelligence and self-expression. They must develop and honor their own internal stress barometer and speak up when they feel overwhelmed or need help, while honoring colleagues who are striving to do the same even though they may need different kinds of help at different times.

COMBATING STRESS WITH SELF-CARE AND COMMUNICATION

The nursing profession is not a good choice for people who cannot handle at least some stress. In fact, a little bit of stress can be a good thing, although what constitutes a "little bit" varies among individuals and over the course of a day and lifetime. According to Paul Rosch (n.d.), chair of the American Institute of Stress, "[i]ncreased stress results in increased productivity—up to a point, after which things go rapidly downhill" (para. 5). This is powerful reasoning for developing self-awareness, honoring needs, and practicing self-expression—in other words, increasing your emotional intelligence and improving your communication skills.

To combat stress, the first step is identifying feelings of anxiety, fatigue, or excessive stress, and the second is asking for help, setting limits, and delegating tasks. Following are examples that illustrate these steps:

- "I need 10 minutes to collect myself. That doctor screaming at me shook me up."
- "Can you help me with this new IV pump? I was stressed during that in-service and didn't take it all in."

Consultant Commentary

Ebright (2010) believes the lack of understanding about the complexity of RN work contributes to limited progress in patient safety. Indirectly related to this essential point is the recognition of how our own well-being is affected by cognitive stacking. We must learn to gauge when we are getting overwhelmed before we make mistakes or become victims of too much stress, and we need to appreciate the effect it has on our colleagues.

In 2011, I had the opportunity to present a workshop on the use of theater games to build communication and collaboration skills in healthcare professionals at the New York University Forum on Theatre for Public Health. During the workshop, I experimented with an activity called "overload" that was intended to develop listening skills. But as I was watching it play out, I was excited to see the possibility for some additional powerful teaching moments. The activity requires four people: one in the center with a person on both sides and one directly in front. The individual in the center is required to count to 100 by fours, all while answering simple math questions and personal questions asked by the two colleagues on both sides and while following the physical movements of the person standing in front of her. It seemed to me that this activity was a way to make visible or substantiate what happens when people are bombarded with interruptions. It helped to demonstrate how very intelligent and highly trained people, like nurses and doctors, can make seemingly foolish and sometimes catastrophic mistakes, such as amputating the wrong leg or giving someone the wrong medication.

I knew I had to capture these teaching moments because they would help us to have compassion for ourselves and each other, improve patient safety, and provide an educational resource for consumers and healthcare professionals. I decided to offer a free workshop to local nurses and students in exchange for participants allowing the event to be filmed and made public. Five nurses and two nursing students participated, and the result is a 12-minute video called, "Interruption Awareness: A Nursing Minute for Patient Safety" (Boynton, 2012). Watching it, you will see how in less than a couple of minutes of participating in the activity, one nurse has trouble answering what her favorite color is and another nurse struggles to add 5 plus 2. These are smart, capable professionals, yet simple questions quickly became profoundly difficult in the midst of chaos—much like the mistakes we make are due to the phenomenon of cognitive stacking. Participating in this "overload" activity could help shed more light on the subject and demonstrate to nurses why they should set limits sooner, ask for help, and avoid interrupting colleagues or making assumptions when stressed.

I'm grateful to the small group of nurses, students, and friends who collaborated to bring this idea to fruition. To date, it has been seen in more than 40 countries and has been viewed more than 11,000 times, and a growing list of healthcare organizations are using it in training. I'm very proud of this grassroots effort to improve patient safety, self-awareness, and nurse workplace settings.

- "I can't work overtime safely tonight. I'm exhausted."
- "Would you get Ms. Yanuka's stat blood transfusion started for me? I'm overwhelmed and need to clarify this morphine order right away so that I can get Mr. Dambuski's pain under control. His wife is a nervous wreck."

A level of stress is involved in all of these scenarios, but emotional intelligence and effective communication keep the stress from becoming harmful. As mentioned earlier, stress can be motivating. Many nurses can remember giving their first injection as a stressful experience. But wanting to do it right for the patient and to pass a clinical expectation is a motivating type of stress that promotes study and practice. When the reward is great, some stress can be beneficial, such as when participating in a life-saving surgery, easing a patient's pain on the medical-surgical floor, answering a birthing partner's questions in labor and delivery, and teaching a student how to give an injection.

Structured communication patterns offer another strategy to manage stress. Such models, including the GRRRR (Greeting, Respectful listening, Reviewing, Recommending or Requesting [More Information], and Rewarding) model detailed in Chapter 3 and the Situation, Background, Assessment, and Recommendation (SBAR) communication model discussed in Chapter 4, may have an added benefit of ensuring accurate transmission of messages during stressful situations. In *Beyond the Checklist: What Else Health Care Can Learn From Aviation Teamwork and Safety*, Suzanne Gordon, Patrick Mendenhall, and Bonnie Blair O'Connor (2013) discuss the idea that predictable communication patterns among pilots and crew during a crisis help to decrease the mental energy being spent on trying to figure out what others are thinking, saying, and expecting. Students should recognize that structured communication models presented in *Successful Nurse Communication* and elsewhere provide clear expectations and opportunities for practice so that, when under pressure, less time and energy will be spent on ambiguity. This will help to decrease stress and allow more focus on the crisis at hand.

CASE STUDY

Janet is a 36-year-old oncology certified nurse who works full time in an outpatient cancer center. She had been working 24 hours per week for 5 years but started full-time work just 6 months ago. When she got the offer, she had mixed feelings because she didn't want to give up involvement in her children's school or cut back on going to the gym. But because she loves work and her husband had recently taken a pay cut in his job, she accepted the position. For the first 3 months, her work performance was excellent. However, that has changed. She now comes in late and calls in sick. She has put on weight and recently had a needlestick injury. In just the past 2 weeks, two young patients died whom she was quite close to. Her colleague found her crying in the break room several times this past week. She has told him she is fine and can handle things, but he is worried about her.

Discussion Questions

1. List all the stressors that Janet might be experiencing. Comment on any ways that emotional intelligence or effective communication could help the situation.

2. Do you think Janet might be suffering from burnout or compassion fatigue? Support your reasoning.

3. What recommendations do you have for Janet for managing her stress?

SUMMARY

Making self-care a priority is critical for all nurses. Nurses' health and stress levels are influenced by many interrelated individual and organizational factors. Self-awareness is an invaluable component of emotional intelligence that can help individuals identify if and when stress is a problem; self-worth and assertiveness are both important to ensure seeking out and accepting support. Gaining experience and confidence are also individual factors that can help to decrease stress. Organizational factors such as staffing will influence how effective nurses are and how good they feel about the care they are providing. It is essential for nurses to seek out ways to nurture their own physical, emotional, and spiritual well-being. They can also encourage colleagues to do the same. Any time there are human factors to consider, the importance of speaking up and listening is fundamental to individual, team, and organizational success. Healthier individuals make up healthier teams, and healthier teams make up healthier organizations—all of which contribute to safe, cost-effective care, optimal patient experience, and rewarding careers.

Reflection Questions

1. Recall a clinical situation in which you felt stressed. Write a paragraph or two about the situation and how you were feeling. In retrospect, do you think cognitive stacking was part of the situation? Was there any time during the situation when you could have asked for help? Do you think you would ask for help during a future stressful situation? Why or why not?

2. Make a list of self-care strategies you already follow and a list of those you should or would like to try. Looking at your lists, consider what factors do or would help you to be successful and what barriers might hinder your success.

3. Write assertive statements that demonstrate what you need and want with respect to self-care.

4. What are two action steps you can take this week to improve your self-care efforts?

5. Think of a colleague you could offer positive feedback to about his or her self-care and then offer it.

References

American Holistic Nurses Association. (2014). Don't burn out—discover self-care and self-awareness. Retrieved from www.ahna.org/Membership/Member-Advantage/Self-care

American Nurses Association. (2001). *NursingWorld.org health and safety survey*. Warwick, RI: Cornerstone Communications Group. Retrieved from www.nursingworld.org/DocumentVault/HealthSafetySurvey-2011.pdf.

American Nurses Association. (2012, February 7). ANA survey: Improved work environment, more can be done. *American Nurse Today*. Retrieved from www.theamericannurse.org/index.php/2012/02/07/ana-survey-improved-work-environment-more-can-be-done

Boyle, D. A. (2011). Countering compassion fatigue: A requisite nursing agenda. *OJIN: The Online Journal of Issues in Nursing, 16*(1), Manuscript 2.

Boynton, B. (2012). Interruption awareness: A nursing minute for patient safety [video]. Retrieved from www.youtube.com/watch?v=PGK9_CkhRNw. [*Author's Note*: Permission to use the video is gained by writing to this author at beth@bethboynton.com; there is no fee.]

Burke, R. (2000). Workaholism in organizations: Psychological and physical well-being consequences. *Stress and Health, 16*(1), 11–16.

Ebright, P. (2010). The complex work of RNs: Implications for healthy work environments. *OJIN: The Online Journal of Issues in Nursing, 15*(1), Manuscript 4. Retrieved from www.nursingworld.org/MainMenuCategories/ANAMarketplace/ANAPeriodicals/OJIN/TableofContents/Vol152010/No1Jan2010/Complex-Work-of-RNs.html

Gessler, R., & Ferron, L. (2012). When caregiving ignites burnout: New ways to douse the flames. *American Nurse Today, 7*(4). Retrieved from www.americannursetoday.com/article.aspx?id=8980&fid=8916

Gordon, S., Mendenhall, P., & O'Connor, B. B. (2013). *Beyond the checklist: What else health care can learn from aviation teamwork and safety.* Ithaca, NY: Cornell University Press.

Lucian Leape Institute. (2013). *Through the eyes of the workforce: Creating joy, meaning, and safer health care.* Boston: National Patient Safety Foundation. Retrieved from http://www.npsf.org/?page=throughtheeyes

Maslach, C., & Jackson, S. E. (1996). *Maslach burnout inventory manual* (3rd ed.). Palo Alto, CA: Consulting Psychology Press.

National Institute for Occupational Safety and Health. (1999). Stress ... at work. NIOSH Publication Number 99-101. Retrieved from www.cdc.gov/niosh/docs/99-101

Rosch, P. (n.d.). What is stress? The American Institute of Stress. Retrieved from www.stress.org/what-is-stress.

Snow, C., & Willard, D. (1989). *I'm dying to take care of you: Nurses and codependence—breaking the cycles.* Redmond, WA: Professional Counselor Books.

Organizations and Successful Nurse Communication

Part III introduces students to organizational concepts in which the application of a behavioral approach to communication is essential. First, students will study organizational culture and the implicit and explicit rules that lead to healthy and unhealthy cultures. Next, students will explore fundamental stages of and current strategies for team development as well as examine the major properties of complex adaptive systems. Finally, students will learn about the exciting role nurses have as change agents in quality improvement efforts as individual and organizational behaviors become integrated into healthy learning organizations.

CHAPTER 9

Understanding Organizational Culture

LEARNING OBJECTIVES

- Describe how communication, emotional intelligence, and behaviors differ in healthy versus toxic organizational cultures
- Discuss the negative consequences of cultures of blame and of bullying
- Describe a culture of safety in terms of behavior and interactions among staff
- Discuss the importance of accountability within a just culture
- Explain how explicit and implicit rules affect organizational culture

KEY TERMS

- Organizational culture
- Toxic culture
- Explicit rules
- Organizational cynicism
- Implicit rules

Organizational culture pertains to how and why things are done in the workplace and the rules that guide them. Organizational cultures can be healthy or unhealthy, and the rules that inform them can be explicit and implicit. This chapter explores the interrelationship between organizational culture and communication practices, emotional intelligence, and behaviors as well as the impact on patient safety, workplace morale, and patient experience. These concepts are an important part of culture change, which will be discussed later in Chapter 12.

THE SIGNIFICANCE OF ORGANIZATIONAL CULTURE

Organizational culture permeates all activities in the workplace. Individual behavior and communication influence organizational culture, and vice versa. There are team, department, or unit cultures that may or may not be compatible with the cultures of other teams, departments, or units of the same organization. Ideally, an organization's culture will be positive and consistent throughout.

The way people interact, how things get done, and the feelings that are evoked in observers are all by-products of the organizational culture. In an ideal healthcare organizational culture, individuals are giving their best; teams are functioning with the clear and common purpose of providing safe, quality care; and everyone has the resources and tools to be successful. Communication, emotional intelligence, and behaviors among staff are demonstrated by the following:

- Open, honest, and respectful exchange of ideas
- Requests for and offering of help
- Timely and compassionate response to patient needs and requests
- The setting of limits and honoring of others' boundaries
- An exchange of constructive feedback
- Ownership of mistakes and willingness to teach and learn

On the other side of the spectrum, a **toxic culture** refers to any culture in which poor behaviors and lack of effective conflict management are part of the day-to-day workplace dynamic. There are many ways that human beings can be disrespectful and avoid or mismanage conflict. In the book *Toxic Nursing* (2013), Cheryl Dellasega and Rebecca Volpe offer a variety of common vignettes and expert commentaries to expose, discuss, and teach strategies for addressing many conflicts and disruptive behaviors that most seasoned nurses have experienced or witnessed. These stories, typical in many nurse practice settings, include topics such as bullying, gossiping, cliques, incivility, and gender bias, and they demonstrate a creative and destructive range of disruptive behaviors and alternatives to healthy conflict resolution. Cultures of blame and bullying are two types of interrelated toxic cultures and are discussed later in this chapter. Conflict management will be explored in Chapter 15.

Organizational culture will be reflected in the first impressions that patients, families, and visitors get when they walk in the door. Behavior, whether good or bad, sets a tone for expectations and tolerance. In a healthy organizational culture, a nurse will stop to help a patient's family find the cafeteria while on her way to the laboratory. A new nurse who witnesses this learns that this is the way patients' families are treated, even if the patient is on a different unit. The priority for helping visitors navigate the hospital environment whenever possible is part of the organization's culture. Conversely, in a more dysfunctional culture, a nurse may walk right by a patient's family and, instead of stopping to help, will continue a conversation with a colleague. A new nurse observing this situation learns that it is acceptable to ignore families in common areas. Both instances reflect the cultures of the organizations: One is engaging and helpful, whereas the other is not.

In both scenarios, emotional intelligence and communication are reflective of the type of culture. In the first instance, the nurse, consciously or subconsciously, uses emotional intelligence to assess the family's confused or distressed nonverbal cues and practices assertive communication in asking if they need help. She may have simply made eye contact, slowed down, and said, "Hello" while approaching the family, giving off receptive body language that the visitors perceived as a welcoming invitation to ask for help. As a result, the family receives the message that the staff cares about them, which is reassuring in terms of how they believe their family member is being or will be taken care of.

Such subtle yet powerful messages are also present in the second, less helpful situation. The nurse may have avoided eye contact, kept her back or shoulder toward the family while approaching, continued her private conversation, and picked up her pace, all of which wordlessly tell the family she is very busy and not available to help. An assertive and empowered family member may interrupt them regardless, in which case the outcome might be the same (i.e., they find the cafeteria), but the family would not infer a message of helpfulness and caring.

A healthy culture will also breed respectful work relationships throughout the organization. In a positive workplace culture, professionals can ask for or give input because they trust they will be respected and they know that learning is an ongoing expectation. Interactions in such cultures contribute to the healthcare professionals' wealth of knowledge and improve their critical thinking skills and moment-to-moment decision making. People in this type of organization are busy, but there is an overall sense of camaraderie and interdependence.

In a toxic culture, colleagues tend to ignore each other as much as they can or align with some colleagues while excluding others. There may be slamming of doors, muttering behind backs, and other passive-aggressive behaviors that suggest a lack of cooperation, teamwork, and mutual respect. The difference between a healthy organization culture and a toxic one is palpable.

Confident Voices

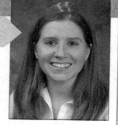

Rebecca Volpe, PhD
Professor and director of Clinical Ethics Consultation

If It Looks Like a Duck, Swims Like a Duck, and Quacks Like a Duck, Then It's Probably a Communication Breakdown

I was initially drawn to medical ethics because a difficult, knotty ethical dilemma is my idea of a good time. To my surprise, when I arrived at my first full-time job after graduating with my doctoral degree, as coordinator of the Clinical Ethics Consultation Service at a large Level I trauma facility, I discovered that at least a third of the ethics consultation requests circled largely around failures of communication.

One such consultation request came within a month of beginning my new role. The bedside nurse called the Ethics Consultation Service and told the following story: "The patient is a 67-year-old lady with a past medical history significant for essential thrombocytopenia and recently diagnosed acute myeloid leukemia. She was admitted last week after presenting to the ED following a fall at home. A CT scan revealed subarachnoid hemorrhage, which does not require any intervention at this time. The patient's family asked me to call you guys. I guess what happened is that the physicians were talking with the patient, and the patient indicated that she wanted to be full code. Almost immediately following that discussion, the family said that they didn't think the patient's expressed wishes to remain full code were commensurate with what they believe to be her long-standing values. Apparently the family feels strongly that the patient would *not* want to be resuscitated given her underlying terminal illness. But the doctors say that the patient had decision-making capacity when she expressed her preference to be full code and that they need to go with the most recent preferences of the patient. But the family is adamant that's not what the patient would want! And the doctors are adamantly against a DNR/DNI code status. Help!"

Confident Voices—cont'd

The core conflict in this case is between the physicians, who believe the patient wanted to be full code, and the family, who believes the patient wanted to be DNR/DNI. The easy fix would have been to simply speak with the patient again and clarify her goals of care, but unfortunately her mental status had declined and she was no longer capacitated.

On the surface, this may not seem like a communication issue. Although there are absolutely ethical issues at play here—most prominently patient autonomy, decision-making capacity, and surrogate decision making—the ethical issues did not *cause* this problem, and resolution of the ethical issues will not *solve* this problem. The cause—and solution—of this consult rests largely with communication.

Let me be specific. The family *simply didn't believe* the physicians when they said that the patient was capacitated at the time of her declaration of wanting to be full code. The family's evidence was ample: Family members could give multiple examples of why they believed the patient would not want to be resuscitated, recounting several episodes during which the patient expressed a desire "not to end up like" other family members who had suffered a serious illness.

Simultaneously, the physicians trusted their *own* experiences (i.e., the bedside discussion when the patient said she wanted to be full code) and were skeptical of the family's reports of the patient's preferences.

Both parties became entrenched in their own view and couldn't see past their own perspective. The bottom-line: A lack of trust between the family and the physicians resulted in significant communication lapses.

Trust is an essential element in communication. A physician and nurse can only communicate effectively if they have a basic level of trust in each other. The same is true for the care team and the family—as we demonstrated in this scenario. And yet trust in healthcare is by no means automatic: Trust has to be earned and can be easily jeopardized.

In my years running the Clinical Ethics Consultation Service, one thing has become very clear to me: Investing scarce clinical time developing relationships— developing trust—is *never* wasted time.

Biography

Rebecca Volpe, PhD, is assistant professor of Humanities at the Penn State College of Medicine and director of Clinical Ethics Consultation at the Milton S. Hershey Medical Center. Dr. Volpe earned her PhD from Saint Louis University's Center for Health Care Ethics and went on to complete a Clinical Ethics Fellowship at California Pacific Medical Center. She is the author, with Cheryl Dellasega, of *Toxic Nursing: Managing Bullying, Bad Attitudes, and Total Turmoil* (2013, Sigma Theta Tau International).

TYPES OF ORGANIZATIONAL CULTURES

There are many types of both healthy and unhealthy organization cultures. Following are short descriptions of the most common.

Culture of Blame

A *culture of blame* is a type of toxic culture in which individuals commonly seek to blame others when something goes wrong. This has been a long-standing and problematic mindset in health-care settings. Consider a scenario in which a patient is given an incorrect medication by a nurse. In a culture of blame, rather than exploring what led to the nurse giving the wrong medication, the nurse is blamed without any further investigation. An incident report is likely to be completed and perhaps include documentation that the error occurred because the nurse failed to follow the medication administration protocol. The physician and family would be notified. If the patient's health is unaffected, the nurse might be warned or given a review of the protocol, which would be the end of it. If the patient suffers any harm, the nurse might be terminated or named in a lawsuit.

In a culture of blame, factors such as poor staffing, constant interruptions, disruptive behavior, and administrative issues may remain unaddressed because of an illusion that the wrongdoing was one person's fault. A blaming culture insidiously encourages staff to hide mistakes and pass the blame to others rather than try to understand all the contributing factors. This is a negative influence on ownership and accountability. From a patient safety perspective, cultures of blame keep underlying problems hidden and contribute to slow progress in improving safety. Sometimes blaming and bullying are both present in the same culture.

Culture of Bullying

Tolerance of workplace abuse, discussed in Chapter 7, often takes place in toxic cultures, specifically a *culture of bullying*. Any time that leaders, colleagues, or bystanders don't speak up about abusive or disruptive behaviors, they are passively contributing to this type of culture. Fear of retaliation, lack of clarity about the inappropriateness of certain behaviors, and a real or perceived threat of termination are all organizational factors that may contribute to a bullying culture. For instance, a staff nurse complains to her manager about a colleague who screamed at another nurse for a simple mistake. In a culture of bullying, rather than exploring her accusations further, the manager tells the nurse to keep them to herself. This tells the nurse that bad behaviors are acceptable in the organization.

In a culture of bullying, the bullies may have formal power in a position of status associated with the organization (e.g., a physician or nurse manager) or informal power, which may include knowledge about or experience with a certain procedure, political alignments within the organization or community, or the capacity to generate or limit revenue. Relationships form that are permeated by mistrust, fear, and/or tacit bargaining conditions, hindering the healthy dynamic necessary for collaboration, open and honest dialogue, and honoring expertise and limitations of all parties. Covert agreements such as the following are hard to identify and seldom discussed openly, yet constantly affect day-to-day, minute-to-minute care in a culture of bullying:

- "If you help me, I'll help you."
- "If you do something for her, I won't do something for you."
- "I'll help her, but only as long as she doesn't help him."

As absurd and even childish as such statements may seem, they are the norm in a bullying culture and ultimately interfere with optimal care. For example, a new nurse comes onto a unit and is immediately excluded from support that would help either in care or in becoming comfortable in his new job. The nurse in charge of patient assignments tends to give preferable ones to the nurses who ingratiate themselves to her by doing her favors. The new nurse decides to align himself with her because there will then be a greater chance he'll get help when he needs it. In doing so, the pattern continues.

Bullying is directly related to the sentinel event data discussed in Chapter 5 and workforce abuse in Chapter 7. Students must learn to appreciate the complexity of abusive behaviors with respect to organizational cultures in which dysfunctional power dynamics and relationships erode or prevent healthy collaboration. The antithesis to the cultures of blame and bullying is a culture of safety.

Consultant Commentary

In a coaching conversation I was having with a nursing supervisor of a long-term care facility, she shared a story with me about a certified nurse assistant (CNA) who had been terminated. The supervisor explained that this employee was one of the hardest working aides on the unit and was always trying to do whatever was asked of her, whether by patients, colleagues, other nurses, or management. She also described the aide as somewhat anxious. The CNA had been with the organization for 10 years on the same unit. One day, a wheelchair-bound resident asked the CNA to help move her to the other side of the room so that she could see the television. The CNA was monitoring another patient who required constant supervision because of a history of aggression. Even so, she made the decision to quickly wheel the resident to the other side of the room, and during those few seconds, the aggressive patient attacked another patient. No one was hurt physically, but a family member witnessed the attack and brought her concern to the supervisor. The supervisor contacted the nursing home administrator, who advised her to suspend the CNA; eventually, she was terminated. The supervisor felt bad but also understood the senior leadership's decision. After all, it appeared obvious that the aggressive patient was the priority, and consequently the CNA should not have left him unattended.

During our conversation, I asked the supervisor some additional questions to help shed light on other factors that might have been involved. She explained that the patient requesting help moving had a demanding family and long history of entitlement behavior (e.g., the patient used the call bell sometimes three to five times an hour for things as minor as moving a pillow or taking a newspaper away as well as more necessary requests for help on the commode or pain medication). About a year earlier, a lawyer representing the family had made a formal complaint about care for the patient, and management held a special staff meeting that focused on making sure staff responded to this patient's needs right away. The supervisor also explained that the unit was often understaffed, and one-to-one supervision was never clearly defined or supported in terms of ensuring staffing for the aggressive resident. With the directive not backed up by adequate staffing to provide constant monitoring, an incident was inevitable.

The supervisor explained how efforts to replace staff who called in sick often failed, and it was not unusual for two rather than three aides to care for the 22 patients on the

Continued

Consultant Commentary—cont'd

unit, many of whom needed two staff members for repositioning, bathing, or toileting. Occasionally, there had been times when only one aide covered a shift with help from the charge nurse, and in more than one instance, it was this aide who carried the workload. The supervisor and I discussed how underlying problems such as inadequate staffing, unclear messages about one-to-one supervision, and unrealistic expectations of family and/or leadership may have contributed to the incident. I encouraged the supervisor to consider talking with management about her concerns. She wanted to but worried that it might put her job at risk.

Sadly, with the termination of the CNA, these underlying contributing factors remained invisible and were not addressed. The illusion of preventing future prolems by terminating the aide gave some satisfaction to the family who witnessed the incident—a false reassurance that their family member would now be safer because the irresponsible staff member was no longer a threat. The CNA suffered greatly and most likely has lost confidence in her ability to do her job well, when in reality she worked in an environment in which she did not have the necessary support or resources to do her job properly. The supervisor felt helpless, and from her behavior, other staff learned that the manager would not stand up for them. This situation clearly occurred in a culture of blame.

Culture of Safety

The work done in healthcare environments is often highly technical and hazardous, and there is always the potential for harm to others and for error and catastrophic events to occur. Healthcare organizations should strive to have a superior safety record. To do so, organizations must create a *culture of safety* that includes the following key features described by the Agency for Healthcare Research and Quality (2014):

- "Acknowledgment of the high-risk nature of an organization's activities and the determination to achieve consistently safe operations
- A blame-free environment where individuals are able to report errors or near misses without fear of reprimand or punishment
- Encouragement of collaboration across ranks and disciplines to seek solutions to patient safety problems
- Organizational commitment of resources to address safety concerns" (para. 1)

Communication and collaborative behavior are clearly the cornerstones of a safe culture, as evident in the following scenario: A nurse is double-checking the settings on an intravenous (IV) pump per the facility protocol for IV medications. He notices that his colleague is about to hang a solution of 125 mg of Cardizem in 125 mL of 5% dextrose in water and run the pump at 125 mL/hour rather than setting the rate at 10 mL/hour, which is what the physician ordered. The nurse speaks up immediately: "Sandy, I see a discrepancy. Recheck your entries and let me take another look before starting this drip." The nurse finds her mistake and resets the pump. She is grateful to the other nurse for catching the error, and both nurses agree to report it to the supervisor, who in turn leaves a message for the unit manager. The unit manager decides to look further into the underlying cause of the mistake, and in doing so, discovers that the color-coding formula for IV medication labels, used to distinguish the infusion rate from the concentration and prescription, has been discontinued by the vendor. She brings this to the pharmacist's attention, who apologizes for not seeking nurse input regarding the change and promises to follow up with the vendor to find options for resuming a color-coding process. The near-miss IV mistake in this case became an opportunity for team members at all levels to collaborate and make care safer for all patients.

Speaking up and listening are inherently important in reporting errors, near misses, or concerns about potential safety problems. Mutual respect and collaboration can only exist when everyone feels safe and confident to do both.

Just Culture

Contrary to the punitive climate that is emphasized in cultures of blame and bullying, in a *just culture*, the emphasis is on creating an open and fair environment, encouraging learning, designing safe systems, and managing behavioral choices (American Nurses Association, 2010). A construct of a culture of safety, a just culture deals more specifically with the complicated influences that old hierarchal and/or patriarchal power dynamics have on patient and nurse voices. As will be discussed in Chapter 10, historically physicians have held much higher status than nurses, and nurses have held higher status than nurses' assistants and patients. These differences in status arise from all sorts of complex socioeconomic, psychological, and gender bias perceptions, expectations, and patterns, which contribute to dangerous barriers to patient-centered care and optimal collaboration. However, in a just culture, differences in status are not fueled by unhealthy egos or power dynamics; rather, they are based on level of expertise. Patients, families, and nurses are full partners in healthcare teams and systems.

In a learning module for the Quality and Safety Education for Nurses Institute, nurse leaders Devjani (Juni) Banerjee-Stevens and Sara Horton-Deutsch (2005–2014) explain how social justice relates to organizational justice and also the importance of recognizing the unequal power dynamics in toxic or bullying cultures in order to create a just culture. They suggest, among other things, that making people with less power responsible for equalizing the power presents a paradox that limits progress. This is evident in superficial efforts to build assertiveness in patients through materials that teach the importance of asking questions and voicing concerns to healthcare professionals. Imagine the pressure a vulnerable and anxious patient might feel in reminding a busy and intimidating nurse to wash her hands. The same discomfort is felt by nurses when trying to be assertive with their supervisors. Because speaking up in an unjust culture means overcoming feelings of inferiority, inadequacy, and shame as well as fears of rejection, humiliation, or even job loss, leaders must be more proactive in creating a just environment.

It is also worth considering how those in higher power positions might be affected by power gradients that are infused with unhealthy communication, behaviors, and stunted emotional intelligence. Barriers to assertiveness on one side of the power gradient may be barriers to listening on the other. Insecurities are present among leaders, too, and respectful listening may be impaired because of pressures to always be right or in control along with false beliefs that others, including patients and nurses, have little of importance to say. Creating a just culture out of a toxic one requires a complex paradigm shift of power in which leaders share and in which staff and patients take on responsibility. A loss of power for some and new accountability for others are potentially a little scary for everyone. This shift that senior leaders face is essentially the same phenomenon that nurses face in empowering patients and that patients face in becoming more empowered. Maintaining compassion for each other's experience is necessary for a safe and peaceful shift.

In a just culture, rather than a blame-free mindset, there is an emphasis on accountability. Leaders of such organizations believe that some errors that professionals make are blameworthy and need to be addressed. Accountability is broken down into three different areas, with respective ways of addressing them:

- **Unintentional human error:** For example, a nurse inadvertently grabs and administers the wrong medication because it looks like the right one and was found where the right one usually is. These kinds of errors could happen to anyone and are addressed by providing emotional support and fixing causes. In this situation, the location and the label of the look-alike medication could be changed.

- **At-risk and intentional behavior:** Behavioral choices may arise from bad habits that save time and in most cases don't cause harm. For example, a nurse in a long-term care facility needs to administer medications for a large number of patients at three separate times. She decides it will be quicker to prepare all the medications for the shift for each patient and put them aside. Pre-pouring medications does save time, and presumably there is little to no risk. However, once poured, the medications are no longer clearly labeled, so errors are possible. To solve this problem in a just culture, leaders would seek to understand why the nurse did this and work with her to develop solutions that are supportive, such as collaborating with medical directors to streamline a schedule of administration that allows time for proper administration or decreasing the nurse-to-patient ratio.

- **Reckless behavior:** This behavior is intentional and is done with full recognition and disregard for the risk involved. Not following sterile procedure with dressing changes of a burn victim who is in critical condition would be an example of reckless behavior that the nurse knows can cause serious harm. In this case, leaders of a just culture would take disciplinary action.

Accountability is important in providing safe care and sustaining a commitment to lifelong learning as a nurse professional. Yet, evolving out of the old hierarchal paradigm may require a period of a blame-free practice as nurses become more trusting with risks associated with being more open and honest. In Chapter 12, students will learn more about the culture change process.

Confident Voices

Jim Murphy
Independent Consultant

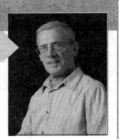

Some Insights Regarding Organizational Culture Change Efforts

Chances are, you are or will be involved in some organizational change effort. Everyone agrees that change is needed in our healthcare system, and initiatives regarding reducing errors, evidence-based medicine, and patient engagement are familiar examples to nursing students. Such efforts generally meet with mixed success and frequently with failure. The chief problem usually is that the changes to be made require altering the organizational culture, whereas the effort was framed about some idea, function, or reform. This is like treating a symptom rather than the cause of a problem.

Confident Voices—cont'd

You can't change the way things are without changing the organizational culture any more than you can reform someone's health without changing the way they think about it. It is in fact very difficult to change organizational cultures, just as it is very difficult to change the habits of people with an unhealthy lifestyle. As you go forward in your career, whatever your level of improvement, understanding the following principles will help you be more effective:

1. **Everyone must be involved.** Everyone contributes to the organizational culture (even if unaware), so everyone needs to be involved if it is to change.
2. **Don't underestimate the effort and resources needed.** In his book, *Leading Change*, the best ever written on the topic, John Kotter (2012) recommends overcommunicating by a factor of 10—in other words, estimate how much communication is needed and then do 10 times that amount. The same can be said of almost every other aspect of culture change.
3. **Be honest about it.** *Are people going to be laid off? What's going to happen to me?* Such questions are endemic in change efforts and needed to be answered honestly. If you are leading the change, you must resist the temptation to temporize and to sugarcoat. If you are caught up in the change, you must insist on your right to honest information, just as a patient has the right to the truth.
4. **Trust and respect are foundational.** Organizations in which staff and leaders trust and respect each other will find change relatively easier, just as cultures that value novelty can change more rapidly. Organizational change, however, usually has to be incremental rather than revolutionary.
5. **Recognize that some people will not change.** Jim Collins (2001), in *Good to Great*, one of the most popular and convincing management books ever, stressed the importance of "having the right people on the bus" and, likewise, of getting the wrong people off the bus. But, just as some patients will not eliminate bad habits, there always will be people who will not fit into the new culture, and it is important that they not be in a position to retard or block the change effort.
6. **Don't make it a campaign with a name and advertising.** Glenn Allen-Meyer's (2000) book, *Nameless Organizational Change*, is not a very well known volume, but it makes a very important point: It is common for change to be "commoditized" and given a name—"Project SMART," say. Not a good idea! An advertising campaign is not the way to change culture.
7. **Support from the top is essential.** It is possible for initiatives stemming from the lowest level to lead to organizational culture change. However, if those at

Continued

Confident Voices—cont'd

the top of the organization are not supportive—and do not model the new behaviors that are called for—it won't work (e.g., the head has to support the new regimen; a patient who is only verbally committed to change won't do it).

8. **Motivation and engagement are the keys.** In *Leading Change*, Kotter (2012) says that there must be a "sense of urgency" (p. 24) to motivate the change. At the same time, he notes that fear is not a good motivator. To overcome inertia, too, excitement is needed. Satisfied patients do better; so do satisfied employees.

9. **Do not suppress, but rather embrace, resistance.** When change is being made, some people are bound to resist. Those leading the efforts frequently look at these "troublemakers" as doctors might look at germs. Indeed, traditional change management literature generally had a chapter on "overcoming resistance." A more modern and better approach is to see resistance as helpful in a diagnostic sense. A sick person may vomit on a doctor, who can then use that substance to determine what the ailment is. Passive acceptance can be even worse than resistance because it means that people are going through the motions but not really on board.

10. **Don't lose hope.** In even the best of efforts, there will be moments when things don't appear to be going well. But it is important not to despair, just as patients are who are too discouraged are less likely to improve. And even when there is outright failure, you can gain from the learning experience.

References

Allen-Meyer, G. (2000.) *Nameless organizational change: No-hype, low-resistance corporate transformation.* Saratoga Springs, NY: Talwood Craig Publishing.

Collins, J. (2001). *Good to great: Why some companies make the leap ... and others don't.* New York: HarperCollins.

Kotter, J. P. (2012). *Leading change.* Boston: Harvard Business Review Press.

Biography

Jim Murphy is a consultant whose focus is on organizational development, change management, and organizational communication. Other specialties include employee surveys, organizational assessments, research, and writing. He has a BS from the Massachusetts Institute of Technology and taught mathematics and economics at several junior colleges. He has been a guest blogger for Confident Voices since 2012, focusing on improving patient experience and healthcare cultures. A proud parent and an avid walker, he lives in Lynn, Massachusetts. Visit his website at www.manage2001.com

EXPLICIT AND IMPLICIT RULES IN ORGANIZATIONAL CULTURE

Almost all organizations have **explicit rules** and goals that provide structure around their organizational vision and mission statements, employee values, norms, and codes of conduct. They are typically visible to staff and visitors in common areas and also found in employee handbooks, employee evaluation tools, and orientation materials. Most explicit rules are set to ensure safe and quality patient care and to provide guidance and expectations about what the organizational culture should be. The nature of the interactions people have and the ways that they get things done are the manifestation of what the culture is.

Formal leaders, including the executive board members, chief executive officers (CEOs), and chief nursing officers (CNOs), play an important role in creating explicit rules, engaging employees to contribute to them, holding staff accountable for following them, and modeling practices. Senior leaders set the stage for everyone's behavior and should at least be perceived to have the authority to enforce the rules. Therefore, these leaders have both the power and responsibility to ensure that the mission, vision, and values of the organization are upheld and that conduct is respectful of all others, always.

Supervisors, managers, and charge nurses also have the power and responsibility to promote and enforce explicit rules, but this can be challenging if the senior leadership is not doing so consistently. When leaders at the top are not able or willing to promote and enforce these rules, mixed messages are sent and double standards may become apparent. For example, a CEO who dismisses a CNO's request for additional nurse staffing is contributing to a mixed message about the organization's commitment to patient care. Granted, this is an oversimplified example because staffing is extremely complicated, but nevertheless, it raises questions among staff about the organization's true purpose and creates doubt regarding other proposals made by the CEO. Such questions and mistrust contribute to **organizational cynicism**, defined as "an attitude arising from a critical appraisal of the motives, actions, and values of one's employing organization" (Bedeian, 2007). In a cynical environment, it is unsafe to be open and honest, and growth in emotional intelligence is stymied. Emotional intelligence becomes a tool for survival used to form alignments rather than opportunities for healthy individual and team growth. Cynicism permeates the culture and shows up in the following counterproductive communication practices and behaviors:

- Ideas are repressed or criticized.
- Requests for help are ignored or ridiculed.
- Response to patient needs borders on unprofessional.
- Limits and boundaries are not respected.
- People talk behind each other's backs rather than providing direct feedback.
- Blaming others is the status quo, and hiding mistakes keeps people in silos.

These behaviors become **implicit rules**—in other words, there is no formal meeting in the conference room to announce them, and they are not written down anywhere, yet many workers follow them. A leader trying to promote and enforce explicit rules can face an uphill battle when implicit rules such as the ones just listed are embedded in the culture.

A frequent instance in which explicit and implicit rules clash is when codes of conduct state "zero tolerance" for abusive or disruptive behaviors, yet tolerance of these behaviors is commonplace in some or all areas. A surgeon who repeatedly humiliates members of the operating room team or a director who ignores reports of horizontal violence without reprimand are role-modeling disruptive behavior. With explicit rules that dictate zero tolerance for disruptive behavior and implicit rules that excuse such behavior, a dangerous gap is created between how the organization proclaims it operates and how it actually does. This creates confusion about what disruptive behavior looks like and makes it very hard to address, especially for those with less formal power.

Such double standards and mixed messages instill mistrust, fear, and blame, which can become pervasive in interactions among all stakeholders. Communication becomes colored by mistrust and infused with invisible limits about to whom and how it is safe to say what. This climate is counterproductive to the open and honest communication necessary for learning, accountability, and ultimately safe care.

CASE STUDY

Mark is excited to begin training as an emergency department nurse. On his first day, the nurse training him makes multiple negative remarks about the physician on duty: "Don't ever make a suggestion, or she'll ream you out. You have to walk on eggshells around her." Later, another nurse is showing Mark where the supplies are kept. She tells him, "If you can't find things, don't call Central Supply because they'll get on your back about wasting resources. It's better to keep a few key things like IV start kits hidden so you can grab them when you need them." Toward the end of his shift, a nurse assistant tells Mark a patient is vomiting violently in one of the examination rooms. However, Mark walks in to find the patient sitting up smiling and only a small amount of emesis in the basin. He hears muffled laughter coming from the hallway. Later in the shift, the nurse who is training Mark comments, "Hope you don't mind a little kidding around. This job can get to you, and it's good to laugh when we can." The remainder of his training is free of other incidents and, overall, goes well.

Discussion Questions

1. What kind of a culture best describes this department based on the scenario? Support your reasoning.
2. What appear to be the implicit rules of the emergency department of this organization?
3. How could Mark use respectful communication to optimize his relationships with the Central Supply staff, the nurse assistants, and the nurse training him? What barriers might exist in building respectful dialogue?

SUMMARY

A culture of safety and a just culture are examples of progressive organizational cultures that support continual learning and foster a climate in which communication and behavior are based on trust. Open, honest, and respectful dialogue is ongoing in these cultures, and these cultures are a sign that healthcare systems are shifting away from old patriarchal or hierarchal workplace cultures in which people of lower status have been intimidated, ignored, or treated unfairly. People in such toxic organizations have had limited power to change things because negative implicit rules have become embedded in the organization's culture. Such implicit rules promote passive or passive-aggressive ways of interacting that interfere with individual and team performance and compromise the delivery of safe, quality care.

Reflection Questions

1. What do you think are the important differences in working in a just culture versus a culture of bullying? In a culture of safety versus a culture of blame?

2. How do you think you would feel if you overheard several of your colleagues talking about another nurse in a negative way? How might this influence the workplace culture, and what could you do to help build a safe and just one?

3. Have you ever experienced a physician or other leader saying something humiliating to you? How did it feel, or how do you think it might feel, to be treated this way?

4. How would you feel about yourself, your colleague, and your career if you shared an experience with a colleague and were told, "You better get used to it. That's the way it is here."? What step or steps could you take that would contribute to a safe and just culture?

References

Agency for Healthcare Research and Quality. (2014). Safety culture. Retrieved from psnet.ahrq.gov/primer.aspx?primerID=5

American Nurses Association. (2010). Position statement: Just culture. Retrieved from nursingworld.org/psjustculture

Banerjee-Stevens, D., & Horton-Deutsch, S. (2005–2014). Cultivating a culture of justice in nursing education and healthcare (Learning Module 13). Retrieved from qsen.org/faculty-resources/modules/learning-modules/module-thirteen

Bedeian, A. G. (2007). Even if the tower is "ivory," it isn't "white": Understanding the consequences of faculty cynicism. *Academy of Learning and Management Education, 6*(1), 9–32.

Dellasega, C., & Volpe, L. R. (2013). *Toxic nursing: Managing bullying, bad attitudes, and total turmoil.* Indianapolis, IN: Sigma Theta Tau International.

CHAPTER 10

Collaboration and Team Development

LEARNING OBJECTIVES

■ Describe the five stages of team development
■ Describe challenges to teamwork common in nurse practice settings
■ Explain how knowledge of the stages of team development can be used to improve collaboration among healthcare professionals
■ Discuss core concepts of teambuilding strategies
■ Discuss the impact that historical hierarchy has on communication and collaboration

KEY TERMS

■ Team development
■ Crew resource management
■ TeamSTEPPS
■ Historical hierarchy

Effective teamwork in healthcare is an essential component of a healthy organizational culture, and it requires followership and leadership from all staff as well as patients and families. Patients receive the best care at the hands of a team of professionals and paraprofessionals who offer different strengths and areas of expertise. In this chapter, students will be introduced to the stages of team development along with the basic leadership and followership needs associated with them. Students will then examine factors that make team development unique and challenging in healthcare settings as well as learn strategies for optimizing teamwork. In addition, students will explore how hierarchy poses a challenge to the collaboration and communication necessary for optimal teamwork.

HEALTHCARE TEAMS

In healthcare, there are many teams working to provide patient care. For example, a primary nurse on a medical-surgical floor is part of each patient's healthcare team, the team of nurses that make up the unit, and possibly a separate team of nurses that typically work on a particular shift. Nurses also work as team members in the organization, and there are teams of people working on committees and in human resources, central supply, maintenance, and other departments.

Teams are characterized to a great extent by their goals, norms, membership roles, and expertise. The various experts on a healthcare team must follow their own scope of practice, licensing requirements, and individual job descriptions. At any minute, a new member may be called on to step in and must be able to seamlessly become part of the active team while another member steps back. Often there is a hierarchical order (discussed in more detail later in this chapter) to healthcare teams that infuses power gradients into relationships and provides a structure to activities. Other rules that govern team conduct include explicit and implicit organizational culture rules (discussed in Chapter 9) as well as any standards that the team itself has agreed to abide by and those built into team development strategies such as TeamSTEPPS and crew resource management, which will be discussed later in the chapter.

Teamwork in healthcare can be complicated for many reasons. Healthcare is a vastly complex system with many variables and very high stakes. Members of the team come from different educational paths, have varied knowledge bases and degrees of experience, and are responsible for a range of specialized and often urgent tasks. Although the primary goal is always to provide safe and quality care, there are often organizational tensions (e.g., budgetary concerns, staff shortages) and various agendas (e.g., filling beds, preventing readmissions, minimizing hospital stays) that pull professionals in different directions. There also may be clinical differences of opinion, such as when to provide comfort measures versus aggressive treatment or when a patient does not want to receive treatment that the healthcare teams believes he or she should.

Team membership varies with staffing patterns, including shift work, weekends, and on-call assignments. Typically, teams are made up of 6 to 24 people, but there can be more or less. Some teams are transient, such as first responders, whereas others have a more permanent existence, such as the nurse management team of a hospital.

Healthcare teams are also influenced by factors including diversity, fatigue, emotional intelligence, training, experience, and the quality of interprofessional and interpersonal relationships. In the face of all these differences, the ability of a team's membership to collaborate and manage conflict is essential for superior results in terms of patient safety and patient experience.

STAGES OF TEAM DEVELOPMENT

Because of the complexity inherent in many healthcare teams and the difficult dynamics that can result when team development is ignored, gaining awareness about the stages of small group or **team development** is critical for students and practicing nurses. Learning about the stages can help nurses make general assessments about where their teams are in the process and what they might need in terms of leadership and followership in order to move to the next stage or remain productive. In addition, as nurses become better able to identify team needs and helpful interventions, they will help to raise awareness about related problems and solutions throughout their organizations.

In the mid-1960s, Bruce Tuckman (1965), psychologist and pioneer in studying group dynamics, theorized four stages of team development: norming, storming, forming, and performing. In the late 1970s, with psychologist Mary Ann Jensen, Tuckman (1977) amended these to include a final stage: adjourning. These five stages have been studied, debated, and tweaked by organizational behavior theorists and business management leaders over the years. Although there is considerable variation in the language used to describe them, their fundamental theories have remained intact.

The first stage, *forming*, occurs when the team initially comes together. At this stage, individuals may be curious to meet others in the group or reconnect with colleagues they have worked with before. They want to learn more about the goals, expectations, opportunities, and challenges. At this point, while the members of the team are functioning independently with a focus on how the team may benefit them or what they might offer the team, there is a sense of connectedness through a shared commitment of being on the team. Team leaders at this stage can help most by giving clear goals and expectations, facilitating introductions among membership, and being accessible and visible in their role. They should be willing to answer questions and hear concerns. Followers are dependent on leaders and are typically curious, excited, and/or anxious about their role and status in the group. They should listen to leaders and others' introductions, share appropriate information about themselves, and ask questions. There is not much conflict at this stage because people tend to be on their best behavior as they get to know each other, although exceptions exist when members bring previously unresolved conflicts into the group (Tuckman, 1965).

Storming is the second stage and, as the name suggests, is full of conflict, tension, and struggle. The team starts to look more deeply at the objectives, and members begin to challenge each others' perspectives and possibly those of leadership. Individuals may be competing for status or approval. Conflicts about roles may arise along with disagreements about priorities. High-stress levels, constraints on time, toxic cultures, and lack of communication skills all provide challenges during this stage. Add to these influences constant change in team membership, lack of awareness of and resources for team needs, and variables in expertise, and it is no wonder that teamwork is often fragmented and problems with collaboration and communication are so pervasive in root causes of sentinel events. During the storming stage, team leaders should remain visible and accessible, and they should continue to portray an authoritative demeanor while creating opportunities for others to speak. Team members need to know who is really in charge; without clear and consistent goals and expectations, they may not fully commit to the work. Leaders should allow some room for conflict related to the group's work, at the same time keeping a sharp eye out for old conflicts that are exacerbated during this time; the former is a healthy natural part of team development, whereas the latter is not. Unresolved conflict and unclear leadership are a combination that can keep groups stuck in the storming stage indefinitely. Leaders can help by asking or even insisting that old conflicts be put aside or by aiding in resolving them; followers should attempt to resolve their own conflicts and be careful not to get caught up in those of others (Tuckman, 1965).

Norming is the third stage, during which members begin to identify as part of the team. Members have agreed to take on the challenges and goals before them, which prevails over bickering or competing for attention. Trust and mutual respect are growing, and differences are appreciated. Although it is not the end of conflict, disagreements tend to be more productive, with resolution being more in sync with the mission of the group. During this stage, team leaders can take on a more collaborative demeanor because group members have begun to rely on each other and themselves. Everyone in the group is actively engaged. There is an increased sense of belonging and readiness for doing the work they have been convened to do, which leads perfectly to the next stage (Tuckman, 1965).

The fourth stage, *performing*, is an exciting, creative, and productive stage that leaders and members find very rewarding. Ideas flow freely and are normally critiqued without judgment or defensiveness. This co-creative collaboration leads to new ways of thinking, which is favorable for team objectives that require problem-solving or new ideas. It is as if everyone were bringing their best selves to the team. Experimentation with ideas is encouraged by leaders, and team members are willing to help each other be successful. It may be hard to distinguish leaders from followers because everyone is contributing and learning. The goals of the group are being met, and there may even be some sadness that the wonderful energy and relationships that have formed soon will no longer be needed (Tuckman, 1965).

Adjourning, the fifth and final stage, is about completion and closure. There may be apprehension and a sense of loss in terms of belonging and purpose, relief that the demanding work is over, and celebratory feelings over the team's accomplishments. These feelings are all natural, and leaders can help by making room to honor successes and say good-bye (Tuckman & Jensen, 1977).

These stages can occur over any length of time, from the course of one procedure in the emergency room to a 3-year culture change process by a management team. Let's consider how the stages would play out during a typical shift: A few minutes are taken at the beginning of the shift for forming to make sure team members know who everyone is, who is in charge, what their patient care assignments are, and any potential concerns. If the team has worked together before, storming may be brief because members are aware of each other's communication skills and clinical competency; however, some discussion about conflict around assignments, organizational changes, or patient concerns may take place. The nurse in charge should listen, validate, and answer any questions in order to move the team to the norming stage, where the group is ready and inspired to go to work. Ideally, the team will be in the performing stage throughout the shift. Finally, the team can take a few minutes at the end for adjourning, even if it is as simple as offering feedback in a postshift huddle.

It can be challenging to apply an understanding of these stages of group development to the real world of nursing, in which there are endless emergent tasks to attend to and constant change. Concerns about thorough team development are easily overlooked and seen as relatively unimportant when nurses are faced with urgent clinical priorities. As well, teambuilding work, such as conflict management and constructive feedback skills, is hard to practice. Yet the underlying dynamics that keep groups stuck in conflict or interfere with their progression through team developmental stages are counterproductive to collaboration and patient safety. In addition to raising awareness and promoting discussion among nurses and nursing students about what is needed to support healthcare teams, here are some scenarios in which nurses can aid in or improve team development:

- A nurse team leader in her report with other team leaders addresses an ongoing conflict: "I would like to have Cara and Robert as the nurse assistants on my team again today. Yesterday, they had a conflict about caring for Mrs. Smith. Since she is still here, I'd like to take the opportunity to work through their conflict."

- An assistant nurse manager shares with his manager his concerns about the unit's recurrent conflicts: "I think our team is stuck in the 'storming' stage of group development. It might be helpful to provide clarity about our goals and to reinforce performance expectations at our next staff meeting."

- A nurse manager in a meeting with human resources suggests a teambuilding opportunity: "I'd like to create a process in which all nurses rotate through alternate shifts periodically or as part of orientation. This will help to build relationships and collaboration among staff on different shifts as well as some empathy for everyone's various demands."

In applying team development steps to nurse practice settings, there must be recognition that, theoretically, every time someone new joins or leaves the group, the team development process begins again. New hires, shift and census changes, vacations, and sick calls alter the makeup of the group and thus present endless and sometimes unrealistic demands for team development in the minute-to-minute dynamic world of 24/7 healthcare. However, there may be creative ways to optimize team development even when the group composition changes often, such as standardizing communication, considering team makeup when scheduling staff, sharing responsibility for clear goals and expectations with leaders and consistent team partners, and including basic information about team development in educational and orientation programs. Additionally, when several new people join the group, there is a new leader, the goals change, the team experiences a traumatic loss, or serious conflicts persist, making the time for more concentrated teamwork is worthwhile. Encouraging team development keeps the importance of teamwork on everyone's radar and should lead to better work relationships, easier and more productive conflict management, improved team performance, and ultimately safer care.

Confident Voices

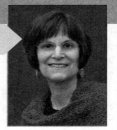

Suzanne Gordon
Journalist and Patient Safety Expert

Team Intelligence and the Pursuit of Genuine Teamwork
There has never been more talk about teams and teamwork than there is today in healthcare. Despite all the talk, there is very little action that helps people learn how to effectively work on teams or what they need to do to make teams work. Indeed, the discussion of teamwork and teams tends to be dominated by explorations of the concept of emotional intelligence with little understanding that emotional intelligence is only part of the story.

If nurses are to learn how to communicate both intra- and interprofessionally in order to deliver quality care and make patients safe, it will be necessary to move beyond concepts of emotional intelligence and teach people how to create and enhance what I call *team intelligence*. Developing team intelligence is critical—particularly to solve the unacceptable crisis in patient safety and to create a more respectful and satisfying workplace.

What do I mean by team intelligence? Team intelligence is the active capacity of individual members of a team to learn, teach, communicate, reason, and think together, irrespective of position in any hierarchy, in the service of realizing shared goals and a shared mission.

Team intelligence involves an understanding of a number of critical concepts and helping people build a toolbox of skills that allows them to create genuine teamwork. In most healthcare workplaces, however, the lack of team intelligence means that people do not work on real teams but are instead intimate strangers involved in parallel play at the bedside.

Confident Voices—cont'd

One of the key concepts that underpins team intelligence is what Edwin Hutchins (1995) calls *socially distributed cognition*. As Hutchins defines it, "[a]ll divisions of labor, whether the labor is physical or cognitive in nature, require distributed cognition in order to coordinate the activities of the participants. When the labor that is distributed is cognitive labor, the system involves the distribution of two kinds of cognitive labor: the cognition that is the task and the cognition that governs the coordination of the elements of the task" (p. 176).

This means that people who work on teams not only have to learn how to do their own work but must also appreciate the value, meaning, purpose, and relevance of the activities performed by the others who work with them. This, in turn, involves the recognition that, no matter what their position in the healthcare hierarchy, people who work in healthcare are constantly using their minds to organize their work and do it effectively. Contrary to conventional wisdom, the highest status players on the healthcare stage, such as the physician or advanced practice nurse, are not the only ones who think critically and make strategic decisions. RNs, LPNs, nursing assistants, housekeepers, unit clerks—to name only a few—also think about their work as they do it. Even though the proverbial buck may not stop with them, they nonetheless have a stake in the outcome of the work of the entire team or group.

Another concept central to team intelligence is that of psychological safety. In their book, *Personal and Organizational Change Through Group Methods*, Edgar Schein and Warren Bennis (1965) argue that those who work together must "unfreeze" if they are to learn new behaviors and work together on teams. Essential to unfreezing is the creation of psychological safety within a particular group so that people can take chances without fear and with sufficient protection: "Learning new ideas and behaviors requires a sticking-one's-neck-out-without-reprisals attitude, as distinguished from playing it safe. Thus a climate is created that encourages provisional attempts and tolerates failure without retaliation, renunciation, or guilt" (p. 44–45).

In a psychologically safe environment, people feel they can ask a "dumb question," stop the line, or challenge a superior about safety without fear of retaliation, humiliation, or disregard. If emotional intelligence encourages leaders to listen, team intelligence goes much farther by encouraging leaders to solicit the input of others—particularly those who are not considered to be high-status players. When leaders have team intelligence, one of their main tasks is to create a psychologically safe environment and, in doing so, encourage people to speak up and welcome their input.

Team intelligence involves many more conceptual leaps as well as building and practicing many more skills as people learn both to lead teams and be assertive

Continued

Confident Voices—cont'd

team members. For the patient to really be at the center of care, those who surround the care must learn to work together effectively and respectfully. Team intelligence can help build the kind of intra- and interprofessional education and practice that make the delivery of healthcare safer for both patients and those who devote themselves to patient care.

References

Hutchins, E. (1995). *Cognition in the wild.* Cambridge, MA: MIT Press.

Schein, E. H., & Bennis, W. G. (1965). *Personal and organizational change through group methods.* New York: Wiley.

Biography

Suzanne Gordon is an award-winning journalist and author who writes about healthcare delivery and healthcare systems and patient safety. She is the author of 17 books, the latest edited with patient safety physicians David L. Feldman and Michael Leonard and titled, *Collaborative Caring: Stories and Reflections on Teamwork in Healthcare* (2014, Cornell University Press). She is also coauthor of a play about team relationships in healthcare, *Bedside Manners.* Gordon is a certified TeamSTEPPS Master Trainer and has lectured all over the world on healthcare issues. She is also a visiting professor at the University of Maryland School of Nursing and assistant adjunct professor at the University of California at San Francisco School of Nursing. Learn more at www.suzannegordon.com

TEAMBUILDING STRATEGIES

Many healthcare organizations seek help from organizational development and leadership consultants to optimize team performance, improve customer satisfaction, and/or promote creativity. Teambuilding may include simple gatherings such as a pizza party and more in-depth consulting work involving assessment, recommendations, and interventions aimed at improving teamwork. More extensive teambuilding activities might include meetings with senior leadership and managers, interviews with staff, facilitated group feedback sessions, focused retreats, and customized training to build trust and communication skills and to facilitate the development of and commitment to norms. Sometimes professional coaching is provided to help resolve conflicts, build leadership skills, or work on especially troublesome interpersonal dynamics.

The healthcare industry is one of many industries, including nuclear power and air travel, that have a lot to lose from ineffective teamwork. Indeed, all healthcare entities can be considered high-reliability organizations, which are those in which high-risk work is performed safely and consistently over time. In healthcare, with the growing awareness of the need to collaborate effectively in order to provide safe, quality service with high reliability, developing teams has become an even more pressing concern. In this vein, two teambuilding strategies are receiving increased attention in the healthcare field: crew resource management (CRM) and Team-STEPPS. Both have arisen to some extent from successes in making air travel safer. They promote psychological safety, healthy hierarchies, positive work relationships, and effective communication, all of which are necessary for optimal teamwork. CRM has a longer history and is built on a general concept that offers some essential lessons for the healthcare industry. TeamSTEPPS was developed as an extension of CRM and is a more standardized, well-defined program; it continues to develop and gain use throughout the United States. Students will likely be exposed to one or both of these strategies as part of the orientation process during clinical rotations or later as they begin their practice as licensed professionals. Specific uses, program variations, and training methods vary depending on the affiliated organization's adaptations and preferences.

Crew Resource Management

Crew resource management (CRM) is an approach to optimizing teamwork and leadership that focuses on ensuring safety in high-risk industries. CRM was originally developed in the aviation industry (in which it was initially referred to as *cockpit resource management*) in the late 1970s and early 1980s in response to an alarming pattern of airline tragedies that seemed to be linked to poor communication and behaviors among the team members and leaders (i.e., pilots and crew).

In their book, *Beyond the Checklist: What Else Health Care Can Learn From Aviation Teamwork and Safety*, Suzanne Gordon, Patrick Mendenhall, and Bonnie Blair O'Connor (2013) describe several airline accidents and subsequent safety investigations that took place during this time. They conclude that "[h]uman interventions could have prevented these accidents and human failures ended up being their ultimate cause" (p. 21). One of the incidents the authors cover occurred in 1978 when United Airlines Flight 173 ran out of fuel and crashed 6 miles from the airport in Portland, Oregon. Out of the 189 on board, 11 passengers and two crew members were killed and 23 people were seriously injured. According to the authors, "[t]his incident became a defining moment in commercial aviation, a tipping point that captured the attention of aviation safety experts and agencies throughout the industry.... [The crash] focused a very bright light on a culture that, while purposeful in the past, had become increasingly dysfunctional. . . . Put very simply, the airline crew culture in 1978 was extremely hierarchal and autocratic" (p. 16). Given the safety problems, high-risk work, and hierarchal structure that make up healthcare, it makes sense to wonder if some of the problems in healthcare have similar roots to those in aviation in the 1970s.

In response to the increased data implicating human error as the cause of crashes, the aviation community turned to psychologists John K. Lauber and Robert Helmreich "to develop new kinds of psychological training for flight crews" (American Psychological Association, 2014, para. 2). This training evolved to include group dynamics, leadership, interpersonal communication, and teamwork and became known as CRM. Over the years, many airlines developed CRM programs using the following core principles:

- Communication
- Workload management
- Teamwork
- Technical proficiency (Gordon, Mendenhall, & O'Connor, 2013, p. 40)

These principles support the behavioral approach to communication taught in this book and reinforce the importance of speaking up and listening as essential skills for effective teamwork. CRM also promotes psychological safety through the concept that all staff feel safe to voice concerns about workload management and resources (e.g., that there are enough skilled professionals and time to do the work).

CRM was fundamental in shifting the work of aviation professionals from individual to team intelligence, making air travel much safer. Through CRM, the air crew learns to think, decide, act, and learn together. As similar problems with safety and human factors have become visible and persistent in healthcare, these lessons from aviation provide an important foundation for teamwork training needs. In addition, they underscore the value of emotional intelligence involving self and others as presented in Chapter 2. In a literature review of adaptations of CRM use in medicine, Laura Pizzi, Neil Goldfarb, and David Nash (2001) found that CRM in healthcare is worthy of further investigation in areas including the operating room, labor and delivery, and the emergency department. A few years later, the Veterans Health Administration was successful in developing and implementing a medical team training program based on the principles of CRM in 43 of its centers (Dunn et al., 2007). However, CRM's biggest contribution to the healthcare industry may be through its link to the development of TeamSTEPPS.

TeamSTEPPS

TeamSTEPPS, which stands for Team Strategies and Tools to Enhance Performance and Patient Safety, is a standardized curriculum initially developed in the early part of the 21st century through the Department of Defense Patient Safety Program and the Agency for Healthcare Research and Quality (AHRQ) in response to growing concerns about safety issues in healthcare and the need to improve communication and collaboration (King et al., 2008). The program was influenced by how CRM addressed safety problems in the aviation industry, but it is specifically developed for the healthcare industry.

What began as training in 50 facilities has grown into a national implementation program in the United States that includes six regional training centers across the country. The goal of the centers is to create a national network of master trainers, who will in turn offer Team-STEPPS training to frontline providers in hospitals and other healthcare settings throughout the country. It is a government-funded program, so there is no charge to participants beyond covering time, travel, and lodging expenses. A variety of educational materials and tools are available on the TeamSTEPPS website (teamstepps.ahrq.gov) and can be downloaded for free.

The program helps to standardize communication and promote teamwork across disciplines and throughout the nation (AHRQ, n.d.). TeamSTEPPS includes a comprehensive set of ready-to-use materials and a training curriculum to successfully integrate teamwork principles into any healthcare system. There are four core competencies—leadership, situational monitoring, mutual support, and communication—aimed at creating and sustaining a culture of safety. These are taught in a three-phased process:

- A pre-training assessment for site readiness
- Training for onsite trainers and healthcare staff
- Implementation and sustainment (AHRQ, n.d., para. 3)

TeamSTEPPS encourages *huddles* and *debriefs* before and after teamwork, respectively, such as before and after a surgical procedure. This reflects the forming and adjourning stages of team development discussed earlier in the chapter.

Theoretically, using TeamSTEPPS, professionals from all regions will be more prepared to bring their expertise to their various teams wherever they go while learning from others and staying focused on safe, quality care.

Consultant Commentary

While many consultants have expertise in a particular area of content such as pharmacology or wound care, my expertise is in helping people work together more effectively and ensuring that everyone's voice is heard; in organizational development circles, this is known as "group process facilitation." In addition to graduate studies and interning, part of my ability to do this work has been achieved through practicing theater improvisation. I had taken improv classes over the years, both for fun and to develop my presentation skills, and came to realize that these very same activities could help healthcare professionals develop their communication skills and interpersonal relationships. I eventually began to incorporate improv activities into workshops by teaching the principles of improv and discussing its value with respect to communication, emotional intelligence, and collaboration in healthcare.

Not long after incorporating improv into my workshops, I attended the first train-the-trainer course in "medical improv," taught by Professor Katie Watson and Dr. Belinda Fu at the Northwestern University Feinberg School of Medicine (NUFSM). I found out that improvisation had been taught to medical students at NUFSM since 2002 and met several professionals who were using improv in a variety of ways in healthcare. In an article describing her work with medical students, Watson (2011) noted that "some experience improv as a transformative practice, because working to listen, observe, and respond in the moment deepens human capacity in many arenas" (p. 1261).

After nurses learn the core principles of improv, it can be practiced in a learning environment that focuses on the process rather than a theatrical performance. There are an infinite number of activities involving individuals, pairs, and small groups that build concentration, status awareness, listening, spontaneity, critical thinking, and much more. The core principles of improv are as follows:

- **Practice saying, "Yes, and ...":** The golden rule of improv, this means that participants must take what is offered by others and build on it. This requires everyone to speak up and listen.
- **Surrender your plan/co-create:** Participants must build something brick by brick together and in the moment, which is analogous to collaborative work and dynamic exchange of ideas.
- **Avoid questions:** This principle is meant not to dissuade asking questions completely, but rather to encourage assertiveness. By limiting questions, participants must contribute their ideas to an activity wheras asking questions shifts the responsibility onto others.
- **Listen/be present:** Listening and being present are essential in building something with others. Pretending to listen will not work in improv because everything is built on what has been said or done before.
- **Be human:** Mistakes are acceptable in improv. The expectation is to acknowledge them and move on. It encourages lightening up about and owning mistakes. Accountability becomes more prevalent, and relationships take on a new tone of respect and acceptance.
- **Remember that you have everything you need:** Participants must learn to rely on themselves and each other. As participants become more comfortable taking risks, they don't spend as much energy being anxious about being judged.
- **Support each other:** Supporting each other is an inherent objective in all improv activities. It is key in building healthly relationships and counteracting toxic relationships.

Just as CRM and TeamSTEPPS are important teambuilding resources for improving collaboration and making care safer, the core principles and activities associated with improv can contribute to the development of emotional intelligence, critical thinking, and positive interpersonal relationships necessary for successful teamwork.

HIERARCHY AND TEAMWORK

Underlying all teamwork in a healthcare organization is the **historical hierarchy**. Discussed briefly in Chapter 9, traditional hierarchy in healthcare is based on a very old mentality in medicine and society in general: Simply put, men had more power and responsibility in decision making and generally held higher status than women. These ideals were prominent in military and medical models throughout much of the 20th century and became embedded in healthcare structures. With some exceptions, historically physicians have been men and nurses have been women. Although gender roles are changing, in many hospitals and doctor's offices today exists a "command-and-control" hierarchy, in which those on the higher rungs of the ladder—whether men or women—exert authority over those on lower rungs and with communication flowing from top to bottom.

Although such a hierarchy sometimes makes sense in a healthcare environment (e.g., during a cardiac arrest with the doctor in charge shouting out orders to the medical team), this old authority and power dynamic has contributed to some very unhealthy and unsafe limitations on collaboration and delivery of care. All too often authority and responsibility have been falsely accompanied by a sense of superiority, whereas those with lesser authority and responsibility have taken on an unearned sense of inferiority, creating an insidious lack of respect for others by leaders and a lack of self-respect for followers. This lack of respect is an underlying cause of poor communication and toxic relationships in the workplace because respecting others is the key to effective listening and respecting self is the key to assertiveness. Consequently, this power dynamic allows disrespectful communication and behavior to flourish and is very destructive to collaboration and teamwork, leading to the following:

- Nurses who are afraid to speak up or challenge authority
- Physicians who don't know how or when to listen to others' expertise
- Patients who are completely dependent on healthcare professionals for decisions regarding their care

Further, such a hierarchy stifles the emotional growth of those on both ends of the power spectrum. People who have more power incorrectly believe they know more about others' needs and wants than the individuals themselves. Listening is perceived to be a waste of time because those in power already know everything. As a result, they lose opportunities to learn from other perspectives and to build relationships of trust and respect. Similarly, people on the lower end of the power gradient learn that they have little of worth to share and devalue their own perspective and input. It is interesting to note that fragile egos exist in those with feelings of superiority *and* in those with feelings of inferiority.

Moving past these old ways of thinking, behaving, and interacting has required an important shift in teaching nursing and medical students. All healthcare workers must now learn how to become more collaborative leaders and followers as well as how to encourage patients to become more empowered. The new goal is not to eliminate the hierarchy but to make it a healthier one in which there is more sharing of authority, responsibility, and decision making based on expertise, education, and knowledge. In this new paradigm, there will be times when the command-and-control hierarchy will be exercised to achieve the best patient care and challenged when appropriate by any team member.

In this healthy hierarchy, the sharing of expertise, decision making, and accountability within a team requires a balance of leadership and followership in order to offer patients the best care.

Leaders at all levels must know how and when to give, elicit, and take in feedback; build relationships with and among team members; and give orders and provide direction. They also must ensure that the expertise and concerns of all team members are expressed and heard. Followers at all levels must be willing to voice their ideas, recommendations, and concerns; listen to those of others; and know when to act quickly and skillfully within the hierarchy. Forgiveness and patience are essential for oneself and colleagues as new skills and behaviors take shape in this new way of working together.

CASE STUDY

Donna is a circulating nurse in the operating room. She has recently had concerns about a new surgical technician, Raelynn, whose adherence to preoperative scrub protocol Donna questions. Donna has given Raelynn constructive feedback about her technique twice, and both times Raelynn said she understood the appropriate protocol to follow. Donna is not convinced and expresses her concerns to the nurse manager, who says she will look into the matter. That same afternoon Donna and Raelynn are called into a preoperative team meeting before scrubbing up for emergency surgery on a teenager who severely injured both legs in a motor vehicle crash. After giving an overview of the patient's condition and plan for surgery, the doctor asks team members to voice any questions or concerns. No concerns are voiced, and the team goes about their preparation. The operation goes very well, and the doctor congratulates the team on a job well done immediately after surgery. However, a postoperative infection several days later forces an above-the-knee amputation of the patient's left leg.

Discussion Questions

1. What teams can you identify in the case study? What stages of team development can you identify? Support your reasoning.
2. Given your knowledge of team development, what could have been done to promote optimal teamwork?
3. Do you think that a lack of teamwork may have been a factor in the postoperative infection? Explain your reasoning.
4. What are some challenges that the perioperative team faces, and what suggestions do you have for addressing them?

SUMMARY

Healthcare teams are complicated entities that can help or hinder patient safety and job satisfaction. Nurses are on many teams and in varying positions of leadership and followership every day. Their presence on all teams is vital to positive patient care outcomes. Nurses who understand the stages of group development and the impact of toxic power gradients will bring important insights into organizational efforts to improve collaboration.

Reflection Questions

1. How do you feel about being a member of a team? What positive or negative experiences have you had in teams you have been part of?

2. Can you identify any efforts that you made or could have made that might have resulted in more positive experiences? How can you be proactive with these contributions in future teamwork? What steps will you take?

3. Are you more comfortable as a leader or follower? Describe why. What opportunities might there be for you to develop your skills in the alternate choice?

References

Agency for Healthcare Research and Quality. (n.d.). About TeamSTEPPS. Retrieved from teamstepps.ahrq.gov/about-2cl_3.htm

American Psychological Association. (2014). Making air travel safer through crew resource management. Retrieved from www.apa.org/research/action/crew.aspx

Dunn, E. J., Mills, P. D., Neily, J., Crittenden, M. D., Carmack, A. L., & Bagian, J. P. (2007). Medical team training: Applying crew resource management in the Veterans Health Administration. *The Joint Commission Journal on Quality and Patient Safety, 33*(6), 317–325. Retrieved from psnet.ahrq.gov/public/02-dunn.pdf

Gordon, S., Mendenhall, P., & O'Connor, B. B. (2013). *Beyond the checklist: What else health care can learn from aviation teamwork and safety.* Ithaca, NY: Cornell University Press.

King, H. B., Battles, J., Baker, D. P., Alonso, A., Salas, E., ... Salisbury, M. (2008). TeamSTEPPS: Team strategies and tools to enhance performance and patient safety. Retrieved from www.ahrq.gov/professionals/quality-patient-safety/patient-safety-resources/resources/advances-in-patient-safety-2/vol3/advances-king_1.pdf

Pizzi, L., Goldfarb, N. I., & Nash, D. B. (2001). Crew resource management and its application in medicine. In *Making health care safe: A critical analysis of patient safety* practices (pp. 501–509). San Francisco: UCSF Stanford Evidence-Based Practice Center. Retrieved from archive.ahrq.gov/clinic/ptsafety/chap44.htm

Tuckman, B. W. (1965). Developmental sequence in small groups. *Psychological Bulletin, 63*(6), 384–399.

Tuckman, B. W., & Jensen, M. A. C. (1977). Stages of small-group development revisited. *Group and Organization Studies, 2*(4), 419–426.

Watson, K. (2011). Perspective. Serious play: Teaching medical skills with improvisational theatre techniques. *Academic Medicine, 86*(10), 1260–1265.

CHAPTER 11

Complex Adaptive Systems

LEARNING OBJECTIVES

- Discuss the importance of understanding complex adaptive systems
- Describe major properties of complex adaptive systems
- Explain how communication skills are inherent in the properties of complex adaptive systems
- Explain why understanding the complexity of nursing practice is related to making care safer, increasing retention of nurses, and decreasing work-related stress

KEY TERMS

- Complexity science
- Systems thinking
- Complex adaptive systems
- Emergence

The study of complex adaptive systems (CASs), also known as complexity science, involves theories and research from a variety of disciplines, including mathematics, economics, biology, nursing, medicine, and behavioral sciences. It is a relatively new and evolving science, with profound implications for the practice of nursing with regard to patient safety, organizational culture, teamwork, and career satisfaction. In this chapter, students are introduced to CASs, explore their major properties, and examine decision-making processes of nurses as a way of understanding the complexity of nursing work and its relationship with patient safety. Because the field of complexity science is vast, multidisciplinary, and rapidly growing, there are variations in nomenclature and focus of interest. In this book, the purpose is to introduce foundational concepts that have particular significance to the practice of nursing and illuminate their relevance to communication and collaboration.

COMPLICATED VERSUS COMPLEX SYSTEMS

Although **complexity science** is already making its way into advanced nursing studies, there are a variety reasons for introducing some basic concepts much sooner in nursing education. Students who understand the basics of complexity science will be able to understand and contribute to solutions to healthcare problems that are based on **systems thinking**, which leading entities such as the Institute of Medicine (IOM) and Quality and Safety Education of Nurses (QSEN) Institute are promoting. In its report, *The Future of Nursing: Focus on Education,* IOM (2010) advises that competency in systems thinking, along with team leadership, decisionmaking, and quality improvement, "must become part of every nurse's professional formation" (p. 2). The full effect of QSEN competencies to improve the quality and safety of patient care, according to associate professors of nursing and QSEN leaders Mary Dolansky and Shirley Moore (2013), "can only be realized when nurses apply them at both the individual and system levels of care" (para. 6).

In order to begin learning about **complex adaptive systems** (CASs), it is helpful to discuss the difference between the terms *complicated* and *complex* with respect to their use in describing systems. A complicated system is one that is made up of many distinct parts that exist separately and have a cause-and-effect relationship. Such systems can be controlled and are predictable. If one part breaks, the system may fail or have limited function until the part is fixed or replaced. A patient-controlled analgesia (PCA) pump, cardiac monitor, and bionic leg are examples of complicated systems.

A complex system is made up of parts that exist and change in relationship with the other parts and in response to the environment. The individual parts have the ability to adapt and learn, and while doing so affect other parts of the system, which also adapt, learn, and affect the system. Individual parts are related in more of a give-and-take process, in which behaviors are responsive, creative, spontaneous, and often unpredictable. When a complex system is broken or not working optimally, it is more helpful to find ways to enable the parts of the system to adapt, grow, and enhance their relationships in ways that are congruent with desired outcomes rather than to try to control them. An ecosystem, a red blood cell, and the staff in a home health organization are all examples of CASs. Nurses work with many complicated and complex systems.

A PARADIGM SHIFT TO COMPLEXITY SCIENCE

In the book, *On the Edge: Nursing in the Age of Complexity,* Claire Lindberg, Sue Nash, and Curt Lindberg (2008) offer a fascinating discussion about the evolution of nursing and medical sciences, from a mechanistic and linear way of studying systems to the new worldview of complexity science, or the study of CASs. The mechanistic and linear way of thinking arose from Newtonian physics, which assumed that systems could only be understood by breaking them down into parts and studying them separately, and from reductionist philosophy, which considered all systems as nothing more than the sum of their parts. This linear thinking contributed to leadership and management methods like the top-down, command-and-control, hierarchical business structures that most practicing nurses are familiar with. In response, hospitals developed separate departments and instituted a clear chain of command, and discipline-specific educational programs such as medical, nursing, and physical therapy became standard. There was no emphasis on building relationships, individual choice, or sharing perspectives among professionals. Doctors, nurses, and other professionals learned little about each other's expertise beyond knowing who gives the orders and who carries them out.

Several trends in the late 20th century helped to raise awareness about problems associated with the command-and-control approach to healthcare delivery and education. First, a rise in medical errors due to lack of collaboration was found to be related to practicing in a top-down hierarchy in which "silo" mentalities and status-driven power dynamics existed. Second, an onslaught of new information and rapid advances in technology created an environment of constant change. Third, cost-containment efforts, including managed care and utilization review, and budget constraints were forcing nurses, doctors, and others to work at a faster pace. This combination of increased incidences of errors, a steady flow of new information, and decreasing resources was a compelling call to action for healthcare leaders to reevaluate models of healthcare delivery.

The IOM's *Crossing the Quality Chasm: A New Health System for the 21st Century* (2001) provided a landmark resource for looking at healthcare through a new lens, specifically as a CAS, and articulating a vision for a future healthcare system where care would be safe, effective, patient-centered, timely, efficient, and equitable. In Appendix B of *Crossing the Quality Chasm*, author and consultant Paul Plsek (2001) offers an excellent primer, "Redesigning Healthcare With Insights From the Science of Complex Adaptive Systems," that provides a basis for understanding the IOM's efforts to address increasing concerns about safety and quality by looking at problems through this new lens of complexity science. The process of examining systems in this way is often referred to as *systems thinking*.

Student and practicing nurses need to understand the basic principles of CAS in order to contribute to the evolution of ideas and solutions associated with the IOM's vision. Further, because the very nature of CASs is dependent on the quality of communication and relationships among healthcare professionals, patients, and families, nurses must to be committed to practicing respectful communication and collaboration. The value of understanding systems thinking will become clearer as students learn more about CASs.

UNDERSTANDING COMPLEX ADAPTIVE SYSTEMS

As indicated earlier, CASs are made up of elements or agents that are interconnected and able to respond to change in their environment in varied ways. Ant colonies, immune systems, and flocks of birds are all CASs. One way to learn about CASs is to think about or watch one in action. Consider a flock of birds flying toward a feeding area on a windy day. The flock appears fluid while flying in the air—up and down, side to side, forward and back. Moving as a group, the individual birds work together as they adapt to what is going on in their environment at that moment. Their formation is not a rigid shape on a straight path, but rather a fluid shape that stays on course while responding to the wind. Any time there is an increase in wind velocity, the individual birds shift course in such a way that they continue to head in the same direction and stay in their group. Some birds fly a little faster and move to the left; some slow down a little and move to the right. No single bird is telling the other birds what to do. Rather, by sharing the same mission—to eat—and by adhering to a few simple rules—avoid collisions, match the speed of their neighbors, and move toward the center of mass—they are able to stay together and adapt to their environment en route.

The rules are constant but following them allows the birds, individually and as a group, to spontaneously adapt to change in varied ways. There was no planning meeting for anticipating increases in wind velocity, yet they were able to manage the change, work collaboratively, and reach their destination. They are practicing **emergence**, in that their behavior is emerging in response to changes in their environment.

Interconnectedness between teams and within organizations keeps things together, optimizes collaboration, and is achieved through interprofessional communication.

Confident Voices

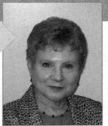

Diana M. Crowell, RN, PhD, NEA-BC
Nursing Education and Leadership Consultant

Animal Spirits and Complexity

I am fully on board with viewing our healthcare organizations as CASs. I find teaching CAS to graduate nursing students absolutely invigorating, and in order to bring it out of the abstract and into the reality of our healthcare lives, I call on some animal spirits to fully make complexity usable in our daily work lives for nurses at all levels. I suggest that as healthcare leaders, we take on some characteristics of the eagle, the ant, and the turtle. Let's look at these three animals and how taking on their behaviors can help us to live and work from a CAS perspective.

The eagle flies high and has a marvelous view and knowledge of the whole territory. The eagle lifts up and out of a situation to see the broader view. Just as an eagle can see around the bend in a river to anticipate what might be ahead, nurses develop the knowledge clinically to anticipate the various scenarios that might unfold for their patients. In the same manner, with astute observation and knowledge of complex systems, you can make sense of the landscape. You can see the nonlinearity, can see that people do self-organize, can see the butterfly effect of one small action on the whole, and can see sensitivity to initial conditions rippling into relationships. And because you can see it and understand it from this vantage point, you can help create the climate for distributed leadership to thrive. With this knowledge, you are not stymied by surprise but see it as part of the process of the system. I often reflect that as nurses we would find our work very dull without some variety to our day. If truth be known, we thrive on surprise and the chance to intervene with skill in relationship with others in order to bring our patients through. I, too, wonder why, when the very same nurses who were adaptable and adroit in handling complex situations are promoted to leadership positions, they become frustrated when things are not predictable but surprising. Furthermore, an eagle knows that there are times when situations are very clear; in such cases (e.g., a state regulation for example), everyone agrees on the course of action, and established linear protocol is the most effective. But other times, there is uncertainty and disagreement as to how to proceed (e.g., whether to expand a department or merge with another organization). We then land in the zone of complexity, that place where a linear solution will not work. This is where Ralph Stacey (2011) would advise bringing diverse people and disciplines together in relationship. This sets the conditions for emergence, or innovative ideas surfacing out of interactions. An eagle knows, too, that things might get messy for a while, but the payoff in idea generation and buy-in is tremendous.

Confident Voices—cont'd

The ant is right down in the workspace, tackling tasks in cooperative relationships with others. The ant perspective is really the linchpin to smooth accomplishment of nursing work and relationships. The ant needs to be focused, present, adaptable, and effective at communicating at all levels. In a medical emergency such as a cardiac arrest—the best example of a CAS—diverse disciplines come together in communication with simple rules balanced and with adaptability as needed.

The turtle is self-possessed and aware and is quite important to our threefold perspective. A turtle is able to stand back, reflect, assess the situation, and ask, "What is happening here? What part might I have played in this drama?" Daniel Goleman's (1995) characteristics of emotional intelligence, self-awareness, self-regulation, motivation, empathy, and social skills are the turtle's best assets.

The trick is to first develop the perspective of each of these animals and then be able to shift gracefully from one to other. In fact, the real goal is to get to the point at which you hold all three in your consciousness at once, or what I consider *embeddedness*: Your turtle is embedded in your ant, and your ant is embedded in your eagle—a cascading effect, a fractal if you will. With the help of your animal spirits, you can be that nurse who forms rich relationships and fosters effective communication with patients and colleagues for the best possible practice.

References

Goleman, D. (1995). *Emotional intelligence: Why it can matter more than IQ.*
    New York: Bantam Books.
Stacey, R. D. (2011). *Strategic management and organisational dynamics: The*
    challenge of complexity (6th ed.). London: Prentice Hall.

Biography

Diana M. Crowell, PhD, RN, NEA-BC, is a national speaker, consultant, and the author of *Complexity Leadership; Nursing's Role in Health Care Delivery* (2011, F. A. Davis). She has served as faculty at all levels of education in clinical and classroom roles, and her administration background includes hospital and educational settings. She leads healthcare teambuilding and leadership workshops in her consultant practice, Leading Your Life, and her greatest delight is bringing energy and new ideas about complexity leadership to her audience. Learn more about her work at leadingyourlife.com.

MAJOR PROPERTIES OF COMPLEX ADAPTIVE SYSTEMS

Exploring properties of CASs is not intended to suggest that healthcare professionals should always be acting without planning or practicing skills; rather, it is to bring into the equation an awareness of the natural human responses to change and the integral elements of communication that are ever present in nursing. Human interactions and relationships are fluid, messy, and surprising. Recognizing that human interactions are unpredictable offers exciting opportunities to influence them in positive ways. Following are descriptions of the primary properties of CASs and how they relate to communication, emotional intelligence, and collaboration.

Butterfly Effect or Nonlinearity

The *butterfly effect*, or *nonlinearity*, refers to an instance in which a small action in one location causes a big impact in another. (The term comes from the theory that a butterfly flapping its wings in one part of the world contributes to a hurricane occurring in another.) Let's consider a scenario in which a nurse overhears a colleague gossiping about her and in response feels hurt and defensive. Later in the day, the nurse decides to sit alone at lunch rather than join her colleagues because the gossiping nurse is among them. She misses a conversation about where the new feeding tubes are located. Later in her shift, she spends extra time looking for a feeding tube, which puts her behind schedule to give another patient pain medication. As she is on her way to give the medication, the patient, anxious and in pain, attempts to get out of bed and falls, fracturing his hip. In this instance, a nurse's gossiping set off the butterfly effect that can be traced to the patient's fall. When humans are the elements of a CAS, the potential butterfly effects are infinite. Using respectful communication is important to minimize negative reverberations and maximize positive outcomes.

Adaptability

Adaptability refers to the ability of the elements of a CAS to respond to and learn from changes in the environment. Sharing information and learning are inherent in this property; for humans, this exchange of information requires assertiveness and listening as well as emotional intelligence, including self-awareness, social skills, and the ability to manage emotions. Adaptability is associated with one's ability to be flexible. Human beings make choices about how they respond to change, and these choices vary with emotional maturity, openness to change, enthusiasm for learning, and a host of other influencing factors. This property is important because rather than imposing or resisting change, both of which stifle adaptability and choice, it encourages nurses to look for ways to empower others or themselves to make healthy choices. Notice how the nurses in the following situations use communication skills to adapt or help others adapt to the environment in positive ways:

- A medical-surgical nurse asks for help from a supervisor who is asking him to pick up a new patient: "Mr. Capelli is nervous and has a lot of questions about his Lovenox injections. I've got a good rapport with him and need more time for teaching. Can you assign the new admission to someone else?"
- A charge nurse looks for the underlying problem with a nurses' aide who is asking for a different patient assignment: "I understand that you are worried about reinjuring your back transferring Mrs. Fletcher. What would help you to feel safer?"
- A nurse at a family practice office talks with a patient whose blood sugars are high and is eating a lot of concentrated sweets: "I understand you are having a hard time limiting desserts after dinner and suspect they may be causing these spikes in your blood sugar at bedtime. Some things that help others include smaller portions, slower eating, and different food choices. What do you think would be most helpful to focus on for you?"

Emergent Behavior

Emergent behavior, closely related to adaptability, describes how the agents of a CAS behave in relationship to others within a particular moment. Nurses are in a continual and dynamic interface with other professionals, patients, and families, and within these interactions emergent or spontaneous behaviors are always occurring. The following examples show how healthcare professionals who practice using respectful communication at all times are influencing emergent behavior or moment-to-moment interactions in helpful ways:

- A day-shift nurse on her way home takes a moment to remind the unit coordinator that the computer system is going to be down during the evening shift.
- A staff nurse overhears a toxic conversation and tells her peers she does not want to talk about another nurse behind her back.
- A housekeeper shares her insight with the clinical team that a postoperative patient's fear of falling was the reason she would not walk with the physical therapist.
- The nurse assistant tells the charge nurse that a new patient is very anxious and unable to sleep, so she wants to spend some sitting with her.

Any and all of these in-the-moment efforts could have easily been missed in an environment where open, honest, and respectful communication is not the norm.

Context and Embeddedness

CASs are frequently embedded within other systems. For example, a unit in a hospital is a CAS itself, but it is also an element of a larger CAS, which is the hospital. The U.S. healthcare system is made up of many other CASs, including pharmaceutical, legal, political, manufacturing, and other related entities. *Context and embeddedness* refers to the fact that the individuals, their teams, the work they are doing, the environment in which they are working, and any related systems all matter. This property can be illustrated by imagining a nurse who is practicing assertiveness and the organizational culture in which she is practicing. If she is speaking up in a culture of respect, she will likely be heard, validated, and thanked for her input, thus reinforcing her assertiveness. If she is speaking up in a culture of blame or bullying, she may be ignored, humiliated, or excluded from social activities, which is more likely to lead to negative consequences such as the nurse leaving the organization or taking on the toxic behaviors. In both cases, the nurse's assertiveness will be felt in infinite ways throughout each system.

Diversity

Diversity can really improve a CAS, in that the more differences that exist, the greater the potential for varied perspectives and creativity. Healthcare systems are melting pots of diversity in every way; variations in age, ethnicity, field of study, religion, and sexual preference are all present. Professionals who respect diversity will be change agents beyond measure because they will tap into creative opportunities that differences offer. Consider how a patient with an above-the-knee amputation following a traumatic motor vehicle crash might benefit from nursing, medical, rehabilitation, psychological, and spiritual expertise that various members of the healthcare team provide. A team meeting to exchange observations and ideas, provided the team is working well together, will improve patient experience. Consideration of the patient's age, gender, primary language, and so on may also contribute to meeting the patient's needs.

Self-Organization

Self-organization is the antithesis of a hierarchical structure and is frequently part of CASs. A good example of self-organization is a group of first responders and volunteers that comes together in the aftermath of major disaster. In *Leadership and the New Science*, Margaret Wheatley (2006) writes about self-organization in response to the tragic events of Hurricane Katrina and the 9/11 attacks: "People who are deeply connected to a cause don't need directives, rewards, or leaders to tell them what to do" (p. 181). Consider a home-health staff nurse who hears about an education program on Reiki in nursing that might benefit all the home care staff and sends an e-mail to several colleagues she suspects will be interested. They, in turn, offer help in finding out more information, raising the possibility with the manager, and engaging with the rest of the staff. This is an example of self-organizing.

One of the key challenges for healthcare leaders and their staff is determining where the hierarchical structure is helpful and where self-organization might work better. Oftentimes, both are needed, such as when responding to a cardiac arrest. The necessary hierarchal events include calling the code, starting cardiopulmonary resuscitation, and getting the code cart. The self-organizing possibilities include comforting a worried spouse while calling for help from an adjacent unit or gathering the response team after the code to acknowledge a failed effort and allowing a few moments for a grieving process.

Simple Rules

As shown earlier with the example of a flock of birds, having a clear vision and a few inherent *simple rules* that the elements of a CAS can follow can lead to desired outcomes. It is worth wondering what healthcare professionals might accomplish if there is a clear and consistent goal, such as safe, quality care, and a few simple rules, such as the following:

- Speak up assertively for patients and self.
- Listen respectfully to patients, colleagues, and self.
- Create a safe and just culture in which speaking up and listening are the status quo.

For example, consider a nurse who is at the end of three 12-hour shifts and receives a request to admit a patient he knows from several previous admissions. The nurse may be tempted to take the assignment because he enjoys the positive feedback of being the "preferred" caregiver or feels pressure to comply with management expectations. However, he is exhausted, and he knows his wife is cooking a special meal and will likely be mad if he is late again. In the old paradigm in which nurses are expected to work overtime and/or do not have the skills to speak up, the nurse might accept the assignment. This might turn out fine, but it might also lead to resentment in the nurse, unsafe care, and frustration from the nurse's spouse. Using the goal of safe, quality care and the simple rules just given, the nurse instead could validate the patient's request while at the same time reporting his fatigue and his desire to be home on time if possible. He might invite dialogue from the supervisor and teammates in which they could brainstorm other ideas:

"I know he trusts me, and I'd like to help, but I'm exhausted. I don't think it is safe for me
    to stay, and I was late coming home last night and the night before," says the nurse.

"I don't mind picking up the admission," his colleague weighs in. "I've been off for 4 days,
    and I could use practice giving IV antibiotics and fluids through the new pump.
    But maybe you can say a quick hello and introduce me to make him feel more
    comfortable?"

In this case, everyone is honored, the collaboration is respectful, and care is more likely to be safe. Also, by giving the patient the chance to develop a new relationship with a different nurse, the team avoids contributing to an unsustainable dependence, and the circle of trusted resources for this patient is widened.

THE COMPLEXITY OF NURSING WORK

The study of CASs helps students appreciate the complexity of delivering nursing care and the implications this has for promoting healthy work environments. This is advocated by the American Association of Critical-Care Nurses (2005) through the following standards:

- "Skilled communication: Nurses must be as proficient in communication skills as they are in clinical skills." (p. 3)
- "True collaboration: Nurses must be relentless in pursuing and fostering true collaboration." (p. 4)
- "Effective decision-making: Nurses must be valued and committed partners in making policy, directing and evaluating clinical care, and leading organizational operations." (p. 5)
- "Appropriate staffing: Staffing must ensure the effective match between patient needs and nurse competencies." (p. 6)

Consultant Commentary

My favorite part of teaching the basics of CASs is watching light bulbs go off as students gain insight into the important and elusive connections between communication skills, relationships, and so many areas of professional practice. There is a sudden clarity about the need to address persistent issues such as patient safety, workplace violence, and burnout with solutions that focus on respectful communication practices and workplace cultures that support them. When students see how a goal plus a few simple rules can work for schools of fish and flocks of birds, they become curious about how the same thing is going on in human systems all around them.

For me, observing CASs is an ongoing curiosity. As part of my self-care regimen, I attend a dance aerobics class. Within it, I see the elements of a CAS. Many people of varied ages, abilities, heights, weights, and skills come together for an hour to dance. We're connected through the music and a commitment to follow the leader. We dance in a very cooperative way that transcends politics, religion, money, age, and ability. The goal is the dance itself, as choreographed by the instructor, and the rules are basically to follows the steps shown and to go in the same direction as everyone else. I find it fascinating to watch how a new move is translated from the instructor and quickly picked up by an experienced few. From there, it catches on throughout the group, as each individual modifies it to his or her own preferences and abilities. Our ability to do this dance is emerging, and as with all human CASs, leadership and followership are going on at all times.

It is exciting for me to bring these same concepts into the early studies of nursing. I truly believe they will influence collaboration and improve care in countless, unpredictable ways.

- "Meaningful recognition: Nurses must be recognized and must recognize others for the value each brings to the work of the organization." (p. 7)
- "Authentic leadership: Nurse leaders must fully embrace the imperative of a healthy work environment, authentically live it, and engage others in its achievement." (p. 8)

Notice how assertiveness, respectful listening, and relationship skills are directly or indirectly related to all of these standards.

Dr. Patricia Ebright leads research that focuses on the complexity of nursing and links it to delivery of care systems, implementing change in systems, and patient safety. In her video, "Complex Adaptive System Theory" (2007), Ebright shows that when a nurse is completing a task, there is much going on that is invisible to an observer. Ebright shares observations made as a nurse manager about how complexity science helped her to understand that everything a nurse is thinking and doing is continually informed, updated, and adjusted by everything else going on:

"If one nurse looks very busy or is getting frustrated with work, it might not be about what they are tuned into right at that moment, but it's about everything that has been going on around the people in the unit and how they're all interacting with one another. Complex adaptive system, complexity theory, is about just that" (1:15). Ebright goes on to connect CAS theory with a story about a nurse trying to explain a frustrating shift to a family member who is not in healthcare and how impossible it is to make sense of it to someone who has not experienced it. Complexity science is a way of making sense of nursing experiences, including all the feelings and decision making that accompany them.

When something goes wrong, such as a medication error or lack of attention to a patient's subtle changes, complexity science brings all elements into question. Rather than blaming the nurse for not following medication administration protocol or critiquing assessment skills, looking at the whole system appreciates that many things were influencing the nurse's decision making. Phone calls and alarms to respond to, changes in staffing and/or patients' clinical status, new equipment being used, admissions, and supplies that are missing or relocated are some things that nurses might need to adapt to. Understanding the complexity of nursing work, according to Ebright (2010), is conducive to promoting four activities that contribute to a healthy (and safe) work environment for nurses (and patients):

- "Designing out" system barriers to care, such as minimizing interruptions and ensuring hand-washing supplies are readily available. This creates a workplace in which nurses can see quickly what is going on around them and have easy access to supplies.
- Designing and implementing appropriate technology, such as ensuring that laboratory results, schedules, and other data are easy to track; simplifying log-in procedures to computer medical records; and providing ergonomic computer stations. A new app that reminds nurses to turn patients is an example of technology that does not take into consideration the CAS world; rather than understand why a patient might not get turned as often as possible, the presumption is that the nurse needs reminding. In reality, patients don't get turned for a variety of reasons, including staffing shortages, time needed for pain medication to work, and a patient's refusal to be turned. Another alarm only adds an interruption.
- Focusing on the direct care function, meaning that the work that nurses are educated to provide should be the priority. Nurses who have to stop to put paper in the printer, duplicate or triplicate documentation, or make the bed for the new admit are not focusing on direct care of patients. Finding out what nurses need to provide safe, quality care is a great way to investigate ways to support their work.

■ **Supporting the new RN,** such as recognition of the learning curve in developing cognitive stacking ability and providing supportive mentorship in the process. It will also be helpful for new RNs to realize that seasoned RNs may not have received such support or awareness of the complexity of their own work.

Ebright's work, along with others who are researching and writing about this CASs, provides an important bridge to the value of communication and collaboration in providing safe care, rewarding careers, and positive workplaces.

CASE STUDY

Karen is a full-time staff RN on a rehabilitation unit at a long-term care facility. She is upset about a new policy that requires staff to punch out for meal breaks and get prior approval from a supervisor for any missed meal breaks. She often skips meal breaks because she believes that the time lost interrupts her flow of work, and she has sometimes missed vital information regarding patients while on meal breaks before. She has been given constructive feedback about time management from her manager. The nurse manager in charge of Karen's unit has been told that she must enforce the new meal break policy because of organizational concerns regarding liability and labor regulations. She makes copies of the policy and hands them out to all staff, telling them that they must comply and to let her know if they have any questions. Karen decides that the best way to deal with this is to punch in and out but continue working. The only nurse she tells is a newly licensed RN, who has indicated that he will do the same.

Discussion Questions

1. What is the rationale for healthcare staff to take meal and rest breaks?
2. What are some possible butterfly effects from Karen's actions?
3. How might leadership use the CAS property of adaptability in order to promote compliance?
4. What opportunities exist for Karen to be assertive and listen respectfully?
5. What ideas do you have for addressing this situation using Ebright's four activities that contribute to a healthy (and safe) work environment for nurses (and patients)?

SUMMARY

Complexity science offers a lens for understanding the interconnectedness, dynamism, and difficulty inherent in nursing practice and patient care outcomes. It reveals how interprofessional communication is important and why nurses must commit to practicing it all the time. This includes learning from mistakes, forgiving self and others, asking for help, offering constructive feedback, appreciating differences, and behaving respectfully even when there is conflict.

Reflection Questions

1. Imagine a situation in which a colleague asks you to help move a patient when you are already overwhelmed with work. What are some possible butterfly effects from helping? What are some possible butterfly effects from not helping?

2. Think about a clinical situation that you experienced as a student nurse that involved a sudden change in a patient's status. How did you and/or others respond? How did this new development affect other things that were going on for you? Did you discuss it with your clinical instructor? How might this have influenced the instructor's plan for the day?

3. What have you observed about the quality of interactions among nurses where you are a student or currently practice? How do you think these interactions might be perceived by patients and families? How are they related to the properties of CASs described in this chapter?

4. How could you respectfully communicate with someone who has different beliefs than you regarding politics, abortion, end of life, or religion?

References

American Association of Critical-Care Nurses. (2005). *AACN standards for establishing and sustaining healthy work environments: A journey to excellence.* Retrieved from www.aacn.org/WD/HWE/Docs/ExecSum.pdf

Dolansky, M. A., & Moore, S. M. (2013). Quality and Safety Education for Nurses (QSEN): The key is systems thinking. *OJIN: The Online Journal of Issues in Nursing, 18*(3), Manuscript 1. Retrieved from www.nursingworld.org/Quality-and-Safety-Education-for-Nurses.html

Ebright, P. (2007). Complex adaptive system theory [video]. Retrieved from www.youtube.com/watch?v=VNFFEJqz9YA.

Ebright, P. (2010). The complex work of RNs: Implications for healthy work environments. *OJIN: The Online Journal of Issues in Nursing, 15*(1), Manuscript 4. Retrieved from www.nursingworld.org/mainmenucategories/anamarketplace/anaperiodicals/ojin/tableofcontents/vol152010/no1jan2010/complex-work-of-rns.aspx

Institute of Medicine. (2001). *Crossing the quality chasm: A new health system for the 21st century.* Washington DC: National Academies Press.

Institute of Medicine. (2010, February). *The future of nursing: Focus on education.* Retrieved from www.iom.edu/~/media/Files/Report%20Files/2010/The-Future-of-Nursing/Nursing%20Education%202010%20Brief.pdf

Lindberg, C., Nash, S., & Lindberg, C. (2008). *On the edge: Nursing in the age of complexity.* Bordentown, NJ: Plexus Press.

Plsek, P. (2001). Redesigning healthcare with insights from the science of complex adaptive systems. In Institute of Medicine, *Crossing the quality chasm: A new health system for the 21st century* (pp. 309–322). Washington DC: National Academies Press.

Wheatley, M. (2006). *Leadership and the new science: Discovering order in a chaotic world* (3rd ed.). San Francisco: Berrett-Koehler.

CHAPTER 12

Change Agents, Quality Improvement, and the Learning Organization

LEARNING OBJECTIVES

- Identify four programs that empower nurses as change agents
- Describe the different models that can be used to achieve quality improvement
- Discuss the five characteristics of a learning organization
- Explain how communication skills and emotional intelligence are necessary to transform toxic cultures and sustain healthy ones
- Discuss necessary steps for organizational culture change
- Identify communication strategies necessary for new nurses beginning practice in an organization in which culture changes are taking place

KEY TERMS

- Change agents
- Quality improvement
- Plan-do-study-act (PDSA)
- Focus-analyze-develop-execute (FADE)
- Learning organization

Change is constant in today's healthcare environment, providing especially rich opportunities for nurses to make positive contributions. Quality improvement efforts are part of the landscape, including revisions of direct care processes, healthcare reform measures that affect financing and access to care, changes in curricula and teaching methods in nursing education, and, most critically, organizational culture shifts from toxic to just or safe. Nurses who practice effective communication and understand their roles as potential change agents will be better prepared for initiating, supporting, and evaluating ongoing quality improvement efforts. In this chapter, students will learn how the role of nurses in quality improvement is evolving, examine the features of a learning organization, explore key principles and importance of creating a safe environment, and affirm the role respectful communication plays all along the continuum.

NURSES AS CHANGE AGENTS

More and more, nurses are being called on to be positive agents of change, or **change agents**, in healthcare systems. The trend arises from growing awareness of safety issues (as discussed in Chapter 5) and the recognition that nurses are by far the biggest workforce, have an indispensable knowledge and skill base, and are present at every interface of the healthcare delivery system. The visibility of this trend became apparent with the landmark report, *The Future of Nursing: Leading Change, Advancing Health* (Institute of Medicine [IOM], 2010). This report addressed concerns about fragmented care in the United States and related problems with safety, quality, and affordability. It resulted in four key messages that revolve around the importance of nurses in creating and sustaining systems that provide safe, quality care to all patients (IOM, 2010):

- "Nurses should practice to the full extent of their education and training.
- Nurses should achieve higher levels of education and training through an improved education system that promotes seamless academic progression.
- Nurses should be full partners, with physicians and other healthcare professionals, in redesigning healthcare in the United States.
- Effective workforce planning and policy making require better data collection and an improved information infrastructure." (p. 1)

The report's primary intent was improving healthcare in the United States, not promoting the nursing profession. As such, it should be noted that illuminating the prominent role nurses have in healthcare and the huge potential for them to have an impact were secondary consequences. Nevertheless, the report represents an exciting call to action for individual nurses, and the profession itself, to take on more responsibility and become more active in all areas of healthcare decision making, from the bedside to the boardroom. This is not to say that nurses have not been responsible or active participants before the report, but rather it notes a shift in the overall awareness and receptivity from healthcare leaders and consumers of nurses' roles in building better healthcare systems and the professional ownership that goes along with it. Many programs are evolving that bring nurses to the forefront of change. The four programs discussed here offer exciting evidence that the voices of professional nurses are becoming more respected and valued.

Transforming Care at the Bedside

Transforming Care at the Bedside (TCAB) was initiated by the Institute for Healthcare Improvement (IHI, 2014) and the Robert Wood Johnson Foundation (RWJF) to improve the quality and safety of care on medical-surgical units by engaging and empowering frontline staff to make positive change. The three-phased program began with three prototype hospitals and grew to include more than 100 hospitals across the United States by the time of its completion in 2008; subsequent efforts, referred to as the *TCAB movement*, have continued to spread to over 200 hospitals. Patricia Rutherford, IHI vice president and TCAB project leader, and Susan Hassmiller, RWJF senior adviser for nursing, oversaw the program. The American Organization of Nurse Executives (AONE) joined the effort in the third phase in order to disseminate the concepts to additional hospitals. Hospital leaders were involved in supporting the project, teams were formed, and nurses were actively involved in identifying problems, generating ideas for solutions, implementing and evaluating new models, and, when successful, spreading those models to other departments. There were originally four goals or themes that the project addressed: safe and reliable care, vitality and teamwork, patient-centered care, and value-added care; a fifth goal, transformational leadership, was added during the third phase (RWJF, 2011).

Following are descriptions of two hospital TCAB projects, including key pilot site activities and qualitative results (RWJF, 2011):

- The Children's Memorial Hospital in Chicago project was "a health and wellness initiative aimed at improving staff vitality. The TCAB unit created a Relaxation Corner—a space for nurses to rejuvenate themselves. The offerings included a massage chair with relaxation CDs, 10-minute neck massages by a therapist, and weekly wellness sessions on such topics as deep breathing and life–work balancing strategies." (p. 48)

- The Kaiser Permanente Roseville Medical Center project "developed special rooms for elderly patients. Called ACE (for Aging Care Environment), the rooms incorporated features to reduce the risk of adverse events to which the elderly are particularly susceptible, especially falls and hospital-induced delirium—which appears to be brought on by medication, the unfamiliar environment and/or other facets of hospitalization. Rubberized, nonslip flooring and special base molding to contrast the floor and the wall for better orientation were two design features. The rooms also had additional tables and chairs to encourage the patient to get out of bed, a VCR/DVD for entertainment and a refrigerator to make liquids readily available and reduce the chance of dehydration." (p. 49)

Other activities that frontline nurses at pilot hospitals worked on included preceptors, rapid-response teams, and educational support for communication (RWJF, 2011). The staff nurses and leaders involved represent an exciting and large-scale investment in engaging direct care staff in quality improvement. The opportunities they had to exchange ideas and apply team-building and systems thinking principles led to better care and more satisfying work. In their overall summation of the project's results, TCAB leaders reported that, "[t]hrough TCAB, a movement has begun to transform the care delivered on medical-surgical units to better serve patients and to transform the work environment to support professional nursing practice and collaborative teamwork at the bedside" (Rutherford, Moen, & Taylor, 2009, p. 17).

There are many resources related to TCAB available at the IHI website (www.ihi.org/engage/ initiatives/completed/TCAB/Pages/default.aspx) that affirm the value of effective communication and empowerment of nurses to optimize quality improvement and provide safe care. Resources engage frontline staff (Rutherford et al., 2008) and optimize communication and teamwork (Lee, Shannon, Rutherford, & Peck, 2008), and include models and processes discussed in this text, such as SBAR and ISBAR (see Chapter 4) and TeamSTEPPS (see Chapter 10). A TCAB toolkit is also available at the RWJF website (www.rwjf.org/en/research-publications/find-rwjf-research/2008/06/the-transforming-care-at-the-bedside-tcab-toolkit.html) for those who want to learn more and integrate processes into their practices.

Clinical Scene Investigation Academy

The Clinical Scene Investigation (CSI) Academy (www.aacn.org/wd/csi/content/csi-landing. content?menu=csi&sidebar=none) originated as a 2-year project funded by RWJF and the Northwest Health Foundation involving seven hospitals in the Greater Kansas City metropolitan area and spearheaded by nurse leaders Karen Cox and Susan Lacey. The academy currently exists as a nursing leadership training program available through the American Association of Critical-Care Nurses (2014). The goal of the project was to involve nurses at the bedside in identifying problems and then have those same nurses drive changes that would solve the issues (Kliger et al., 2010). Nurses involved in the project received coaching and mentoring support. This aided in empowering them to lead changes that resulted in better care, lower costs, and, eventually, the expansion of the CSI program. In one success story, nurses at the Kansas City Veterans Affair Medical Center identified heel ulcers as a problem. Their recommendations included mandatory training on wound/skin care for staff, regular rounds by a wound care specialist, and a weekly "Heels Angels" day to maintain awareness among staff and patients. Their efforts resulted in an 80% decrease in incidence of heel ulcers and an estimated savings of a million dollars or more (Kliger et al., 2010). The CSI project illustrates how leaders can pave the way for direct care nurses to be more involved by ensuring that their voices are respected, that they will be listened to, and that they maintain a high level of clinical accountability. Direct care nurses must be self-motivated and invested in the process.

The Future of Nursing Campaign for Action

The Future of Nursing Campaign for Action (campaignforaction.org) is a national initiative formed to help guide the recommendations of *The Future of Nursing* report (IOM, 2010). The campaign is coordinated through the Center to Champion Nursing in America, an initiative of the AARP, the AARP Foundation, and RWJF (Future of Nursing Campaign for Action, "About Us," n.d.). The campaign promotes ideals for a healthcare system in which all Americans have access to high-quality care and in which nurses are contributing to the full extent of their education and training. This is an encouraging branch of joining consumers and healthcare professionals in programs to ensure access and quality. "Action coalitions" are forming all over the United States and include physicians, nurses, policymakers, business professionals, and others. For example, the Indiana Action Coalition is working on programs to improve inter-professional educational opportunities for healthcare professionals (Future of Nursing Campaign for Action, "State Action Coalitions: Indiana," n.d.). The impetus behind the coalition's work is to improve collaboration and teamwork that are necessary to provide safe quality care. The coalition is co-led by physician Richard Kiovosky and nurse Kimberly Harper. This doctor–nurse leadership team is in and of itself a remarkable shift in sharing governance. Of further note, the coalition's education committee is made up of two doctors and two nurses, and the steering committee includes nurses, doctors, and other healthcare professionals. The opportunities for these professionals to take on new roles and the challenges in doing so will force them to practice their communication skills. It might be out of a nurse's comfort zone to step into an equal leadership role with a physician. The nurse will be challenged to speak up and share her ideas, while the doctor will be challenged to listen more and step back from being in charge.

Quality and Safety Education for Nurses Institute

The Quality and Safety Education for Nurses (QSEN) Institute (qsen.org) was created by the University of North Carolina at Chapel Hill School of Nursing and funded by a grant from RWJF with the "challenge of preparing future nurses who will have the knowledge, skills, and attitudes (KSAs) necessary to continuously improve the quality and safety of the healthcare systems in which they work" (QSEN Institute, 2005–2014, para. 1).

The first of four phases was led by Dr. Linda Cronenwett, dean of the school, and included a panel of 17 nurse leaders. The focus was on defining six key competencies that prelicensure nursing students needed: patient-centered care, teamwork and collaboration, evidence-based practice, quality improvement, informatics, and safety. In the second phase, pilot schools integrated the competencies into their curriculum and QSEN launched its website. In the third phase, the QSEN faculty was joined by the American Association of Colleges of Nursing; its executive director, Geraldine Bednash, became a co-investigator for the project. Together, they developed resources and expertise needed by nursing faculty to teach the competencies. The

Confident Voices

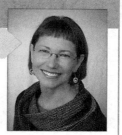

Stephanie Frederick, RN, MEd
Integrated Health Consultant

Finding the Courage and Recognizing Our Worth

A few months ago, I overheard a hospital administrator say he was sending "his" nurses to "smile" school at an associate's hospitality agency. I'm certain he was aware that his hospital had the largest nursing turnover in the community, but perhaps he still wanted to pretend "his" nurses were well treated and generously compensated. A few weeks later, when presenting to a large group of seniors about "How to Advocate and Navigate Healthcare," there was a unified gasp when I informed them that medical errors are now the third leading cause of death in the United States, just behind heart disease and cancer (Allen, 2013; Hospital Safety Score, 2013). *How can that possibly be?* I was asked.

Although nurses have always advocated for their patients, there's been an ethical contradiction about what nurses can share about the quality and safety of patient care in the facilities where they're employed. There are issues such as company operations, unsafe medical practices, poor staffing, and ongoing problems that are consistently reported and not addressed. While the visible message has been for nurses to advocate for patients, there has been an invisible one to protect and serve their employer.

Nurses and patients alike have been assumed to be passive, although we all inherently know we are powerful. With the Affordable Care Act (U.S. Department of Health and Human Services, 2014) in place, there are major healthcare shifts and accountability practices now showing where the dangerous working conditions, inadequate staffing, and organization-wide dysfunctions are occurring. By focusing on the goals of Triple Aim (Institute for Healthcare Improvement, 2014) to enhance the patient experience, reduce costs, and improve population health, the United States will ultimately optimize health system performance. By sharing supportive evidence and collaborating on best practices, a new integrative health model will strive to treat the whole person, support self-care, use less invasive approaches first, and partner with others (Center for Optimal Integration, 2013).

Our voices are needed. Nurses are creative, resourceful, and perceptive. We have expertise, information, ideas, and experience that can benefit everyone. We must recognize our worth and not become too tired or too busy to make our collective voice heard.

Nurse collaboration will become a reality after we first feel and then practice being individually empowered. Have courage in joining together with nursing colleagues

Continued

Confident Voices—cont'd

to offer support. Be unwilling to relinquish basic human rights like nourishment, bathroom breaks, and time off from work. Respect colleagues who have different strengths and limitations. By educating, informing, and advocating for each other, we can remain powerful, active participants in our own self-care. For some nurses, this will be easier than others. Take a long look inside and believe in your worthiness. Here are some ideas that might be helpful:

- Continually seek to lovingly care for yourself. Face your fears, nurture your spirit, and get out and play!
- If feelings are stuffed, they have a way of coming out "sideways" (e.g., through codependency, alcohol and drug abuse, addiction to gambling and shopping, rage). Find the courage to participate in 12-step recovery programs, employee assistance, and other counseling services to help identify the source of pain.
- Learn how to set boundaries in interpersonal relationships. Preserve dignity and self-respect at all costs.
- Engage a personal health coach to assist with building personal and professional communication skills or a psychotherapist for deeper work.

The resulting sense of dignity and self-respect will keep us out of the quagmire of self-destructive behaviors. As a collective force, nurses will continue to be aligned with patients who seek a positive healthcare experience and who want traditional and/or holistic support for their continued health and well-being. Health educators and wellness coaches are examples of how nurses are moving away from a sick care model toward one that truly focuses on sustainable health for everyone.

Although we all realize that there are inherent risks in embracing change and making our voices heard, there are infinitely more risks in having our voices silenced. Ethical oppression will rip out our collective heart and soul. Find the courage to be assertive, collaborate respectfully, and celebrate the intangible gift of nursing.

References

Allen, M. (2013, September 19). How many die from medical mistakes in U.S. hospitals? *ProPublica*. Retrieved from www.propublica.org/article/how-many-die-from-medical-mistakes-in-us-hospitals

Center for Optimal Integration. (2013). Project for Integrative Health and the Triple Aim (PIHTA). Retrieved from www.optimalintegration.org/project-pihta/pihta.php

Hospital Safety Score. (2013, October 23). Hospital errors are the third leading cause of death in U.S., and new hospital safety scores show improvements are too slow. Retrieved from www.hospitalsafetyscore.org/hospitalerrors-thirdleading-causeofdeathinus-improvementstooslow

Confident Voices—cont'd

Institute for Healthcare Improvement. (2014). The IHI Triple Aim. Retrieved from www.ihi.org/Engage/Initiatives/TripleAim/Pages/default.aspx

U.S. Department of Health and Human Services. (2014). Read the law: Affordable Care Act. Retrieved from www.hhs.gov/healthcare/rights/law

Biography

Stephanie Frederick is passionate about empowering, educating, and guiding individuals to become proactive and engaged in their preferred healthcare. In addition to 30+ years as a registered nurse, Stephanie holds an MEd in Health Education. She owns her own business as an independent health advocate and guides clients in receiving safe, quality medical care and additional services that support "whole-person" health and well-being. Learn more at www.stephaniefrederick.com.

fourth phase, launched in 2012, focused on providing educational resources and training to enhance the ability of faculty in master's and doctoral nursing programs to teach quality and safety competencies. Efforts for the fifth phase are being led by Pamela Austin Thompson, chief executive officer of AONE, with the Tri-Council for Nursing, which is made up of the AONE, American Association of Colleges of Nursing, American Nurses Association, and National League for Nursing. There are many learning modules and resources available on the QSEN website that are geared to professors of nursing as well as a new feature called QStudent, which includes an interactive blog for engaging students from different schools in dialogue around related topics (QSEN Institute, 2005–2014).

QUALITY IMPROVEMENT

The importance of nurses being able to share ideas and report concerns, abilities rooted in effective communication, cannot be understated. One area in which nurse input is critical is in the day-to-day delivery of safe care. **Quality improvement** refers to any changes in the delivery of care that focus on doing a better job of meeting the six aims promoted by the IOM (2001): care that is safe, effective, patient-centered, timely, efficient, and equitable. Quality improvement is both a process and an outcome, and all improvements are subject to evaluation and further improvement. Examples of quality improvement include decreasing incidence of pressure ulcers on a long-term care unit, optimizing communication during patient handoffs between the emergency room and the medical-surgical floor, and increasing compliance with hand-washing protocols in a family practice setting. There is extensive literature on quality improvement, and it is accomplished through a variety of models, including root cause analysis (discussed in Chapter 5). Two additional models are discussed here that can be used to introduce quality improvement concepts to students: the rapid-cycle improvement model, also known as plan-do-study-act, and the focus-analyze-develop-execute model.

The **plan-do-study-act (PDSA)** model allows for changes to be made on a small scale so that the impact can be determined quickly. PDSA was made popular by management consultant W. Edward Demings and has its roots in the well-known scientific method of hypothesizing, experimenting, and evaluating (Taylor et al., 2013). Typically, the process begins with three questions:

- What are we trying to accomplish?
- How will we know if a change is an improvement?
- What change can we make that will result in an improvement?

After these questions are asked and answered, the four steps can be implemented:

1. Plan: Plan a change or test how something works.
2. Do: Enact the change or test.
3. Study: Examine the impact the change has.
4. Act: Determine if the change should be modified, abandoned, or expanded.

Although common in healthcare practices, PDSA requires rigorous testing and standardization in order to evaluate its effectiveness (Taylor et al., 2013).

Another common improvement model is known as **focus-analyze-develop-execute (FADE)** (Wiseman & Kaprielian, 2014):

1. Focus: Define and verify the process to be improved.
2. Analyze: Collect and analyze data to establish baselines, identify root causes, and point toward possible solutions.
3. Develop: Based on the data, develop action plans for improvement, including implementation, communication, and measuring/monitoring.
4. Execute: Implement the action plans, on a pilot basis, and install an ongoing measuring/monitoring (process control) system to ensure success.

Both the PDSA and FADE models run in cycles, in that after step four is executed, it signals the start of step one. Duke University offers an online learning module that reviews PDSA, FADE, and other quality improvement models in more detail (Wiseman & Kaprielian, 2014).

Quality improvement can even be developed into a mindset, in that nurses can cultivate it by being alert to how current procedures affect care, staying on top of research, inviting patient feedback, and engaging in dialogue with members of the healthcare team around making healthcare safer and affordable. The quality improvement mindset relies on nurses' ability to express ideas and concerns, and to listen to those of others. Active participation in any process of quality improvement will be more effective if communication is open, ongoing, and respectful. In addition to willingness to participate in ongoing dialogue and processes, for quality improvement to be achieved, the organizational culture of the healthcare facility must be supportive. Safe and just cultures, discussed in Chapter 9, both support the communication and collaboration necessary for successful quality improvement.

THE LEARNING ORGANIZATION

A healthcare organizational culture that embraces both ongoing change and quality improvement is referred to as a **learning organization**. The term was first introduced by Massachusetts Institute of Technology (MIT) Sloan School of Management professor Peter Senge (1990) in his groundbreaking book, *The Fifth Discipline: The Art and Practice of the Learning Organization*. Senge, who was trained as an engineer, had an extraordinary ability to expound and synthesize ideas, resulting in one of the most popular and influential business books of all time.

Confident Voices

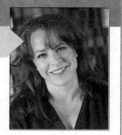

Leilani Schweitzer, BA
Patient Liaison

An Education I Wouldn't Wish on Anyone

I am a healthcare outsider. I do not have a nursing degree, nor have I spent endless hours in clinical rotations. However, the world of healthcare is not foreign to me. My credentials come from experience and observation. My degree comes from an education I wouldn't wish on anyone. And to my outsider eyes, there seems to be endless efforts to improve healthcare. Heaps of good intentions, initiatives, surveys, studies, ideas, and action plans, all leading to more things to do with less time to do them in. Higher expectations and less patience. My outsider status gives me a unique view of the lofty goals, and it allows me to offer ideas to get to the core of the problems facing everyone involved and, ultimately, to the solutions.

Ask for and give help. With limited resources and unlimited demands for time and attention, I imagine there will be many instances when you will need help, and so will your colleagues. Often, solving a problem ourselves is seen as the mark of a good student or employee, but it may also create the possibility for an accident. The night my son died, his nurse asked for help. I learned this detail 9 years after his death. She knew Gabriel was not doing well and recognized he was in terrible pain. She knew that to properly take care of him she needed help. She didn't get it. I wish she had been more insistent and didn't feel the need to do it alone. I wish there had been a safety net to catch both her and Gabriel. I wish she had been helped.

Remember that patients don't want to be patients. With rare exceptions, people do not want to be in hospitals. We don't want to be sick, and when we are with you, we are afraid. Of the days and weeks I have spent in hospitals, despite receiving good care, every moment was colored by a shadow of fear and helplessness. For you as a nurse, being in a hospital is a choice because your career takes you there. It is your place of business. But nothing about it is ordinary or typical for us. We want to meet you at our daughter's ballet class, on a ski hill, or at a neighborhood block party. We do not want to meet you in a hospital. We are there solely because something bad has happened to us. Your work is your job. Your work is our life.

Treat patients as you would want to be treated. When I talk to people about transparency after medical errors, sometimes I get excuses about why it will never happen. I hear explanations about legal maneuvers, complex insurance concerns,

Continued

Confident Voices—cont'd

and resignation that the problem is just too big. But these blocks can be eliminated by considering two questions:

- What would happen at your hospital if a child died because of an error?
- What would you want to happen if that child was yours?

Do not forget your power. You have chosen a career of remarkable influence. Daily, hourly, and possibly every minute of your working day you are affecting the lives of people. That power should not be treated lightly. In the daily, grueling challenges as a nurse, you may forget the impact you have on us, but we are acutely aware of it.

When it was determined Gabriel likely needed surgery, I drove roughly 250 miles from Reno, Nevada, to Palo Alto, California. Our route was complex. It took us over the Sierra Mountains and through San Francisco. Traffic was heavy; we spent 30 minutes parked on a bridge. Gabriel was very sick; his cries sounded like a kitten's. I desperately wanted a helicopter rescue. I was relieved to arrive at the hospital, with no wrong turns and no car troubles. The clock read 7:02 when we parked. The hospital staff knew we were coming, but the nurse was far from welcoming. She did not say hello or ask about the sick child in my arms. After hearing my son's name, her response was, "We expected you at 7:00." Could she have known that 7 hours later Gabriel would die because his brain herniated and that no one would know because an overworked nurse unknowingly turned off the alarms? Of course not. Do I remember the sting of her indifference at the suffering of my son? Yes, nearly 10 years later, I still clearly remember.

I remember the nurse who turned off Gabriel's monitors as well. She was tall, graceful, kind, and a bit frantic. Anyone who looked at her could see she was moving very quickly. Remembering now, she reminds me of a swallow—flying fast, suddenly changing directions. I feel a tremendous amount of compassion for her. I know her life changed, like mine, for the worse when Gabriel died. It all happened without anyone's intention. But her colleagues' decision not to help her was deliberate, and so was the admitting nurse's response to me. Those things happened because of deliberate decisions. And those choices all added up: an admitting nurse who chose procedure over compassion; a room nurse without a voice or system of support; a staff too wrapped up in their own toil to take a moment to help a fellow professional. Deliberate decisions and conscious choices. All unintentionally creating a disaster.

Life is full of complexity and mystery. Healthcare greatly magnifies this truth. It brings opportunities for triumphant successes and abject failures. How you navigate

Confident Voices—cont'd

this truth and how you purposefully treat yourself, your colleagues, and your patients is what will give your career consequence and ultimately richness.

Biography

Leilani Schweitzer did not choose a career in healthcare; rather it chose her. After her son's death nearly a decade ago after a series of medical mistakes, she now works in risk management at the same hospital where those errors happened. As a patient liaison for Stanford University Hospitals, she uses her own experience with medical errors to navigate between the often insular, black-and-white, legal and administrative sides of medical error, and the gray, emotional side of the patient and family experience. Her work at Stanford gives her a unique view of the importance and complex realities of disclosure.

(An updated edition of *The Fifth Discipline* was published in 2006, and two field books were published in 1994 and 1999).

Change and quality improvement are interrelated and involve individuals, teams, and systems; Senge's concept infuses learning ideals in all organizational activities. Learning organizations make a deliberate commitment to ongoing learning, and create systems and processes that promote improvement. According to Senge (1990), learning organizations are made up of five disciplines: personal mastery, mental models, shared vision, team learning, and systems thinking.

Personal mastery is an individual's commitment to the knowledge and practice of his or her profession, going beyond simply "doing a job" to acquiring the characteristics, such as objectivity, detachment, and understanding, and skills for being an expert practitioner (Senge, 2006). A nurse's personal mastery includes a commitment to lifelong learning that is consistent with individual responsibility in quality improvement and contributes to the overall organizational culture. This includes continuing education, sharing ideas, and listening respectfully to others.

Mental models are pictures in one's head of how things work and how that fits into a particular situation. They are based on instincts, beliefs, and theories (Senge, 2006). In a toxic culture, mental models might include staff's beliefs that they will not be treated fairly or respectfully. In a culture of blame, staff would hold a mental model that if something goes wrong, they are likely to be the target of fault. In a learning organization, on the other hand, the mental model is one of trust and faith, and quality improvement is a process in which everyone is engaged with the purpose of finding what truly works best for the safest delivery of care. There is much less, or possibly no, need to be defensive in a learning organization because open and honest dialogue is the status quo.

Shared vision involves common understanding and a picture of how the organization operates and of its future. It is based on an individual's dedication and thus comes from inner motivation rather than external controls (Senge, 2006). Most healthcare organizations advertise a vision statement that promises safe, quality, and compassionate care for all patients, but toxic cultures persist, suggesting that the vision is not shared. In a learning organization, staff are self-motivated to learn and improve systems because they want to be part of an organization that provides such care.

Team learning is the way in which groups collectively figure out together how to work together and achieve needed results (Senge, 2006). It involves the active participation of all team members in thinking and learning together. Open dialogue is a crucial element for healthy team process to unfold and for any quality improvement efforts to be successful in terms of generating ideas, testing them out, and ensuring that changes are communicated to all stakeholders.

Systems thinking involves an appreciation for the relationships and all of the properties of complex adaptive systems (discussed in Chapter 11) in order to understand and influence behavior. It is an exciting concept that builds on the patient-centered care that manifests in a learning organization when all healthcare professionals are working together on a patient's behalf.

Senge's model of the learning organization weaves together the core concepts in this book. Communication and emotional intelligence are critical for effective collaboration and essential for delivery of safe, quality, cost-effective care. Learning organizations in healthcare that have a consistent patient-centered vision, are staffed with highly trained professionals, encourage giving and receiving feedback, and have a culture that supports open, honest, and respectful communication hold much promise for generating new ideas and solutions to all challenges nurses face.

The IOM (2013) publication, *Best Care and Lower Cost: The Path to Continuously Learning Healthcare in America*, goes into great depth in linking quality improvement to organizational culture. The IOM report reviews the 25-year time span from the use of beta blockers following a heart attack in 1982 to the actual common practice of physicians prescribing them in 2007. Although evidence existed to provide best care, the time it took for the knowledge to become common practice resulted in lost opportunities to save lives and improve quality of health. What's needed, according to the report, is an "infrastructure that makes the process of learning and improvement easier, so that the next discovery does not require 25 years of sustained effort before it is used to help patients" (p. 135). The following four characteristics, adapted from the report, describe a continuously learning healthcare organization:

- Science and informatics, which require real-time access to knowledge and digital capture of the care experience

- Patient and clinician partnerships in which patients are engaged and empowered

- Incentives that are aligned to encourage improvement, identify and reduce waste, and reward high-value care and full transparency that makes all information available for fully informed decisions by patients, families, and clinicians

- Continuous learning culture that is stewarded by leadership committed to a culture of teamwork, collaboration, and adaptability, and supportive system competencies and that constantly refines care delivery and provides training, skill building, and feedback loops

The language that the IOM uses differs from Senge's five disciplines; however, the implications for individuals, teams, and complex adaptive systems are similar in that they share a vision of effective communication, empowered change agents, and overall collaborative care.

CULTURE CHANGE

Many healthcare organizations are embarking on journeys to transform toxic cultures to ones that are safe and just and that include continual learning. Consequently, dynamic transformations are part of the landscape in many nurse practice settings.

Culture change efforts, from adapting to new government or consumer expectations to ensuring a mindset of continuous quality improvement, frequently take years to accomplish.

Students may be entering an educational institution, working with clinical partners, and eventually joining a facility where a major shift is just beginning or is already in progress. In response, many nursing schools are working to transform curriculum to better prepare students to serve consumers and to meet the shifting needs and goals of these organizations.

Changing an organizational culture is a major undertaking that requires leaving old perceptions, behaviors, and attitudes behind and developing new ones. Because all healthy cultures are built on effective communication and respectful behaviors, and many organizations have some degree of mistrust among staff, creating a safe environment is an important step in transforming organizational culture. For example, in a culture of blame, staff members are used to being blamed and blaming others when something goes wrong, so there is likely to be fear and suspicion among staff and between staff and leaders. To transform into a just culture, leaders and staff must be willing to stop looking at mistakes as someone's fault and start looking at them as an opportunity to improve a process or equipment. However, changing attitudes and behavior is more complicated than it might seem. A climate of open and honest communication in which assertiveness and respectful listening are the norm must be established first, and giving and receiving feedback must become an ongoing dynamic process. Leaders who are learning to share power and staff members who are learning to take on more power must learn to deal with vulnerability due to perceived risks such as job security and reputation. Although the decision to create a safe or just culture and build a learning organization most likely comes from senior leadership, all levels of staff are integral to the process.

Creating a Safe Environment for Change

There are five key steps that help create a safe environment for effective communication and optimal collaboration. When these steps are followed, everyone has ample opportunity to develop the positive skills and behaviors needed to change organizational culture.

First, a clear and compelling vision about what the new culture or code of conduct is going to look like must be defined. Creating a vision is typically leadership's responsibility to initiate, yet engaging staff from the very beginning is important. For example, an organization's senior leadership team might create a draft statement about respectful communication and behavior to begin a shift in conduct. Brainstorm sessions, newsletters, or surveys create opportunities for staff to be part of the process. If leaders role-model listening with genuine curiosity and intent to use insights, staff members are more likely to be active participants or even champions of the new culture.

Second, acknowledgment must be made of any inappropriate behaviors. A toxic culture breeds mistrust, which contributes to withholding information, defensiveness, close-mindedness about other people's ideas and concerns, job dissatisfaction, and poor morale. Although leaders may be reluctant to focus on negative experiences, finding a way to demonstrate ownership is a crucial step for transforming workplaces into ones where individuals feel safe to reveal imperfections and share ideas. Acknowledging toxicity and apologizing for any perceived and real mistreatment will go a long way toward opening the door to true collaboration. Balancing ownership of the negative with a positive vision of the future will give many mistrusting staff the hope and desire to contribute to the new culture.

Third, explicit and consistent expectations for interpersonal behavior need to be set. As discussed in Chapter 9, both implicit and explicit rules exist, and it is best to have them in alignment. There must be a commitment to organization-wide adoption of respectful communication and conduct. Mixed messages sent through implicit rules (e.g., it is okay for nurses to gossip) or double standards (e.g., abusive behavior by an important surgeon is acceptable) should not be tolerated.

Fourth, initial training and ongoing practice must be considered equally important. Although formal training in communication skills provides an intellectual basis, practicing them is much harder than it might seem. Given the combination of stressful work and challenging behavior changes, creating opportunities for practice is vital. Learning curves will vary with experience, emotional maturity, support system, history, and other variables. There will be times during an emergency when old patterns of disruptive behavior may erupt or defensiveness may occur when receiving constructive feedback. Rather than expect perfection in the messy reality of communication and behavior, it is better to strive for conversations that include ownership, forgiveness of self and others, and a willingness to reflect and consider how others are affected by one's behavior.

Fifth, conduct should be enforced at all levels to send the message that the organization is serious about being fair. There must be a disciplinary process for those who insist on being disruptive, no matter who they are.

Effects of Controlling Cultures

Because transforming cultures requires behavioral changes of individuals, teams, and the complex adaptive systems they are part of, it is helpful to understand what kinds of attitudes exist in a rigid hierarchy. The late Chris Argyris, a pioneer theorist of organizational behavior and professor of education and organizational behavior at Harvard University, wrote many books and articles on these topics over the course of almost 50 years (Smith, 2001, 2013). Argyris believed that overly controlling management leads to passivity and dependency among staff, and that the more mature individuals were, the more frustrated they would be. In his early research, he observed common responses that employees had when coping with frustrations associated with controlling leadership (Argyris, 1957). In subsequent discussion of his work, Lee Bolman and Terrence Deal (2003) note that Argyris found "that employees inevitably look for ways to respond to these frustrations" (p. 121):

- "They withdraw—through chronic absenteeism or simply by quitting." (p. 121)
- "They stay on the job but withdraw psychologically, becoming indifferent, passive, and apathetic." (p. 121)
- "They resist by restricting output [or engaging in] deception, featherbedding, or sabotage." (p. 122)

Consultant Commentary

I use the principles of creating a safe environment as a consultant but also as a per diem RN in a locked dementia unit in a long-term care facility. My job is to ensure a safe environment for all residents. Occasionally, one member of the community may be harassing or bullying another. When one resident yells at another, I will often intervene by sternly telling the person yelling that it is not okay to talk to others like that. If residents cannot understand my instruction or are unable to control their behaviors, the next step is to distract them with another activity and, if necessary, separate them. However, in that moment when I intervene, I am using verbal and nonverbal language to tell the entire community what behavior is acceptable and what is not, and that I am in charge and keeping them all safe. Even many people with dementia will get the message on some level that they are safe and that disruptive conduct is not okay.

- "They try to climb the hierarchy to better jobs." (p. 122)
- "They form alliance (such as labor unions) to redress the power imbalance." (p. 123)
- "They teach their children to believe that work is unrewarding and hopes for advancement are slim." (p. 123)

These responses are reflected in issues such as passive and passive-aggressive behaviors and burnout (discussed in Chapters 7 and 8, respectively). They also help to explain challenges healthcare leaders face in empowering staff and patients. A controlling management can also be linked to the historical hierarchy (discussed in Chapters 9 and 10). In other words, the old power structure has contributed to the development of dependent and resentful mindsets, which are barriers to full participation in healthcare decisions from important stakeholders such as nurses and patients. Suspicion, anger, and mistrust contribute to patterns of passive-aggressive behaviors, especially when assertiveness skills are lacking and there are no channels to express one's voice in a healthy way. If a person or group does not, or perceives not to, have input into a planned change, resisting the change, whether covertly or overtly, is a very effective way of demonstrating power. Furthermore, when people feel powerless, they may lack the desire to develop assertiveness.

HONORING NURSES OF THE PRESENT

Nursing students of today do not ever need to tolerate inappropriate behavior. Coming into the field with compassion, understanding, and respect for their predecessors' experiences can help ensure best outcomes for all.

Although many nurses are excited about changes in the profession and workplaces cultures, some may be resistant to change or disillusioned with their careers. Many seasoned professionals have gained their expertise in the midst of toxic culture stressors such as burnout, compassion fatigue, bullying, and relentless change. A nurse who has worked excessive overtime or has sustained a work-related back injury may resent the profession or her employer. Seasoned healthcare professionals have also likely witnessed much heartache, grief, and tragedy. To deal with feeling frustrated, disrespected, and invalidated, some experienced nurses sadly seek validation by exposing new nurses to some of the toxic behaviors they have endured.

In some cases, it may be best to minimize contact with nurses who exhibit unprofessional attitudes or behaviors, and truthfully it is not another nurse's responsibility to "fix" burned out or disillusioned colleagues. However, there are rich opportunities for new nurses to practice communication strategies that allow for respecting the nurse's experience and knowledge while taking assertive steps to insist on respectful behavior. For example, a new nurse might say to a more seasoned colleague: "I know you have a lot of valuable experience, and I want to learn everything I can from you. However, even though I am new, I expect to be treated respectfully." New nurses can also be intent listeners and perhaps offer another pathway for validation: "It sounds like you have worked a lot of overtime and faced many understaffed shifts in your career. How does it feel when a new nurse comes along and refuses to do the same?" There is no guarantee that conversations like these will pave the way to respectful relationships, and of course the decision to try is a personal one, but making the effort seems worth the potential gains of securing important knowledge and offering compassion for nurses who have spent years caring for others while experiencing toxic behaviors by colleagues, patients, families, administrators, and physicians. One of the challenges that newer nurses face is appreciating and respecting the experiences of their predecessors as well as learning important skills from them, but not engaging in old patterns of disruptive behavior.

CASE STUDY

Maria, a graduate nurse, is very excited about her full-time position on a 24-bed suba-cute rehabilitation unit of a long-term care facility. During her interview process, the director of nurses explained that the organization was beginning a culture change process to eliminate toxic behaviors and that everyone had received training in as-sertiveness and respectful listening. After 3 weeks of orienting to her unit, Maria is given the responsibility of caring for half of the patients on the unit while a licensed practical nurse (LPN) with more than 20 years of experience cares for the other half. Maria has been told by other nurses, including the nurse manager of the unit, that this LPN is a great clinician but often abrupt and that the best way to deal with her is not take her attitude or curt responses personally. Maria has also noted some gossiping among nurses about the LPN, but she does not take part in it. Maria's first few shifts are very stressful for her, but she is anxious to do a good job. There are several times when she has questions and seeks out the LPN's help, but the LPN acts impatient, rolls her eyes, and sighs heavily when Maria approaches her. As time goes on, Maria also notices that the LPN takes meal breaks longer than a half an hour. This is especially stressful for Maria because she is providing care in her absence. Maria is working later than she is supposed to and has had to skip her own meal breaks a couple of times.

Discussion Questions

1. What suggestions do you have for Maria in terms of communicating with the LPN?
2. How would you describe the current culture of the organization? Provide reasoning to support your observations. What are some possible ramifications in terms of patient safety and Maria's career?
3. How could Maria help ensure a successful culture change?
4. How do you think the nurse manager is influencing the culture? Do you have any suggestions for Maria in terms of communication with the manager?
5. How do think you might respond if you found yourself in Maria's situation?

SUMMARY

The effort to create an environment where learning takes place, change is ongoing, and patient care is the focus requires nurses to speak up assertively and to listen respectfully. Regardless of what phase an organization is in, nurses will be called on to be positive change agents all along the continuum, and their success will depend on the clinical skills, knowledge, and attitudes necessary to provide care, including their abilities to be adaptive and to be lifelong learners and teachers.

Reflection Questions

1. Have you ever had an idea about a solution that you kept to yourself? Why might you have done so?

2. What do you find exciting about the future of nursing? How do you see yourself practicing a few years down the road? What examples of lifelong learning have you observed among classroom and clinical instructors and practicing nurses in clinical rotations?

3. Consider an opportunity in which you could be a positive change agent as a student nurse. What ideas do you have that might lead to an improvement in a classroom or clinical rotation? What action will you take?

References

American Association of Critical-Care Nurses. (2014). Clinical Scene Investigator Academy. Retrieved from www.aacn.org/wd/csi/content/csi-landing.pcms?menu=csi&sidebar=none

Argyris, C. (1957). The individual and organization: Some problems of mutual adjustment. *Administrative Science Quarterly, 2*(1), 1–24.

Bolman, L. G., & Deal, T. E. (2003). *Reframing organizations: Artistry, choice, and leadership* (3rd ed.). San Francisco: Wiley.

Future of Nursing Campaign for Action. (n.d.). About us. Retrieved from campaignforaction.org/about-us

Future of Nursing Campaign for Action. (n.d.). State action coalitions: Indiana. Retrieved from campaignforaction.org/state/indiana

Institute for Healthcare Improvement. (2014). Overview: Transforming care at the bedside. Retrieved from www.ihi.org/engage/initiatives/completed/TCAB/Pages/default.aspx

Institute of Medicine. (2001). *Crossing the quality chasm: A new health system for the 21st century*. Washington DC: National Academies Press.

Institute of Medicine. (2010). *The future of nursing: Leading change, advancing health*. Washington DC: National Academies Press.

Institute of Medicine. (2013). *Best care and lower cost: The path to continuously learning healthcare in America*. Washington DC: National Academies Press.

Kliger, J., Lacey, S. R., Olney, A. Cox, K. S., & O'Neil, E. (2010). Nurse-driven programs to improve patient outcomes: Transforming care at the bedside, integrated nurse leadership program, and the clinical scene investigator academy. *Journal of Nursing Administration, 40*(3), 109–114.

Lee, B., Shannon, D., Rutherford, P., & Peck, C. (2008). *Transforming care at the bedside how-to guide: Optimizing communication and teamwork*. Cambridge, MA: Institute for Healthcare Improvement.

Quality and Safety Education for Nurses Institute. (2005–2014). About QSEN: Project overview. Retrieved from qsen.org/about-qsen/project-overview

Robert Wood Johnson Foundation. (2011). Transforming care at the bedside: An RWJF national program. Retrieved from www.rwjf.org/content/dam/farm/reports/program_results_reports/2011/rwjf70624

Rutherford, P., Moen, R., & Taylor, J. (2009). TCAB: The "how" and "what." *American Journal of Nursing, 109*(11), 5–17. Retrieved from journals.lww.com/ajnonline/Fulltext/2009/11001/TCAB__The__How__and_the__What_.3.aspx

Rutherford, P., Phillips, J., Coughlan, P., Lee, B., Moen, R., Peck, C., & Taylor, J. (2008). *Transforming care at the bedside how-to guide: Engaging front-line staff in innovation and quality improvement*. Cambridge, MA: Institute for Healthcare Improvement.

Senge, P. (1990). *The fifth discipline: The art and practice of the learning organization*. New York: Doubleday.

Senge, P. (1994). *The fifth discipline fieldbook: Strategies and tools for building a learning organization.*. New York: Doubleday.

Senge, P. (1999). *The dance of change: The challenges to sustaining momentum in a learning organization*. New York: Crown Business.

Senge, P. (2006). *The fifth discipline: The art and practice of the learning organization* (2nd ed.). New York: Doubleday.

Smith, M. K. (2001, 2013). Chris Argyris: Theories of action, double-loop learning, and organizational learning. Retrieved from infed.org/mobi/chris-argyris-theories-of-action-double-loop-learning-and-organizational-learning

Taylor, M. J., McNicholas, C., Nicolay, C., Darzi, A., Bell, D., & Reed, J. E. (2013). Systematic review of the application of the plan-do-study-act method to improve quality in healthcare. *BMJ Quality and Safety: The International Journal of Healthcare Improvement.* Retrieved from qualitysafety.bmj.com/content/early/2013/09/11/bmjqs-2013-001862.full.pdf

Wiseman, B., & Kaprielian, V. S. (2014). Patient safety—quality improvement: An overview. Retrieved from patientsafetyed.duhs.duke.edu/module_a/module_overview.html

PART IV

Successful Nurse Communication in Action

In order to prepare students for practicing under their own license in the real world, there are three key areas that require additional study: diversity, technology, and leadership. The chapters in this section cover each of these topics as well as provide overviews of conflict and delegation. Although these skills taught here warrant further practice and study, the fundamentals presented will help provide a starting point for students and new-to-practice nurses.

CHAPTER 13

Diversity, Inclusion, and Dignity

D iversity involves the acknowledgment and acceptance of differences in people. What individual nurses think and feel about diverse coworkers, patients, and families, as well as how they behave toward and communicate with them, will influence their ability to collaborate with colleagues and to provide safe, quality, equitable, and patient-centered care. In this chapter, students will learn why diversity is important in nursing and in turn will be challenged to examine their own attitudes about difference. In addition, they will explore how and why respectful communication and emotional intelligence are essential for creating a climate of inclusion in which diversity and collaboration can thrive. Finally, they will delve into the concept of promoting dignity by eliminating rankism.

DIVERSITY AMONG HEALTHCARE CONSUMERS AND WITHIN NURSING

Diversity in human beings is reflected in age, race, gender, gender identity, ethnicity, religion, sexual preference, political values, socioeconomic status, educational background, intelligence, and any other variable that distinguishes one person from another. Because everyone will need to seek healthcare services for themselves or a loved one at some point in their lives, the healthcare consumer pool is literally made up of every type of person. Nurses must have the knowledge, skills, and attitudes to provide care to a truly diverse population. (This is known as *cultural competence* and will be discussed in more detail shortly.)

Although the makeup of the consumer population encompasses all differences, the nursing workforce in the United States is not as diverse. According to the U.S. Census Bureau (2012), individuals from ethnic and racial minority groups account for more than one-third of the U.S. population (37%). Yet a 2013 survey conducted by the National Council of State Boards of Nursing and the Forum of State Nursing Workforce Centers (Budden et al., 2013) indicates that nurses from minority backgrounds represent only 17% of the registered nurse (RN) workforce. Broken down by ethnicity, the survey results show that the RN population is comprised, approximately, of 83% white/Caucasian, 6% African American, 6% Asian, 3% Hispanic, 1% American Indian/Alaskan Native, 1% Native Hawaiian/Pacific Islander, and 1% other; with respect to gender, men comprise just 7% of the RN workforce. In an American Association of Colleges of Nursing (AACN) report for 2013–2014 (Fang, Li, Arietti, & Bednash, 2014a), it was revealed that nursing students from minority backgrounds represent 29% of students in entry-level (also known as *generic*) baccalaureate programs, 30% of master's students, and 28.4% of students in research-focused doctoral programs. In terms of gender breakdown, men comprise 12.5% of students in generic baccalaureate programs, 10.3% of master's students, 11.3% of practice-focused doctoral students, and 8.7% of research-focused doctoral students. With respect to full-time nursing faculty, the researchers note that 13.1% of full-time nursing school faculty come from minority backgrounds: 7.1% black or African American (not Hispanic origin), 2.7% Asian (not Hispanic origin), 2.3% Hispanic or Latino, 0.4% American Indian/Alaskan Native, 0.4% Native Hawaiian/Other Pacific Islander (not Hispanic origin), and 0.2% two or more races; only 5.5 % are male (Fang, Li, Arietti, & Bednash, 2014b).

These statistics and observations about diversity among consumers and within the nursing workforce suggest that working with and caring for people who are different is an integral part of nursing practice. Consequently, nursing students must make it a priority to understand why diversity is important and to develop or sustain positive attitudes toward it.

DEVELOPING A POSITIVE ATTITUDE TOWARD DIVERSITY

There are many compelling reasons that nurses should develop and maintain positive attitudes about diversity. Although more complex than presented here, research and common sense both support the idea that a diverse workforce including nurses from varying ethnic, cultural, and socioeconomic backgrounds can better understand and address health concerns of diverse patient populations. Shared languages, common belief systems, and similar life experiences provide a basis for empathy and respect that can enhance assessment, health education, and overall communication. Diverse professionals can also bring more awareness to the workforce about special needs and challenges that certain populations may have. A special supplement of *Public Health Reports* (Williams et al., 2014) offers substantial proof that health disparities are driven largely by social, economic, and environmental factors and that a diverse workforce is essential to improving health outcomes among minority ethnic and culture groups or populations with socioeconomic disadvantages.

As presented in Chapter 11, diversity is also integral to creativity and innovation in complex adaptive systems, and positive outcomes such as quality and safety are dependent on effective communication and healthy relationships among healthcare professionals and with patients and families. A diverse and cohesive workforce will have more perspectives, new ideas, and better problem-solving capacity.

Nurses have a moral imperative to develop and role-model healthy attitudes toward diversity. This is a world where aggression—arising from differences in political perspectives, religious beliefs, ethnicity, sexual preference, and so forth—toward others is common and sometimes tragic. Given the size of the workforce, long-held trust placed in the nursing profession, the multitude of social and familial interfaces, and the overall commitment to caring for others, there is immeasurable opportunity for nurses to have a significant influence in the world. The valuable impact that nurses may have on local and global communities by promoting positive attitudes toward diversity is outside the scope of evidence-based thinking, sounds lofty, and may be tough to prove. However, despite the uncertainty of this ideal, the vision of a more respectful world is likely to resonate with many nursing students and inspire such a commitment.

Confident Voices

Keith Carlson, RN, BSN, NC-BC
Board Certified Nurse Coach

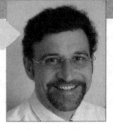

Nurses, Culture, and Communication

Healthcare in the 21st century is an especially collaborative process, and respectful and clear communication creates an environment wherein that collaboration can be most successful. When we communicate with patient and families, the stakes can be particularly high if we are not communicating at the most powerful level possible.

When we consider the notion of diversity in respect to communication, the stakes are raised even higher. In a world where we are faced with multiple languages, beliefs, and cultural practices that may be unfamiliar to us, our ability to communicate effectively can be challenged, as can our own assumptions about what is appropriate or not appropriate when it comes to medical intervention.

No matter the milieu in which nurses interact with patients, our communication with patients and their families is no less important than our communication with other members of the healthcare team. Yes, the content may be different, but the need for clarity and the absence of ambiguity could not be more paramount than when we are attempting to make sure that patients and their families are fully informed healthcare consumers.

Nurses Are Educators

Nurses are natural educators within our scope of practice, and in most circumstances we spend more time with patients than physicians do. Not only do we provide direct patient care in the form of nursing interventions, but we also explain the logic of the treatment plan, the potential outcomes of that plan, and the role that the patient and/or family will play within that crucial process.

Aside from the nuts and bolts of teaching dressing changes and other techniques to patients or their families, we also provide moral, spiritual, emotional, and psychological support. This information must be imparted in a way that is sensitive, appropriate, and free of the cultural bias or assumptions that can easily diminish or confuse the message.

Nurses Are Interpreters

It is often our role to interpret "physician speak" for the patient, distilling a doctor's prognosis or treatment plan in a way that patients can understand. Couple "physician speak" with cultural and language differences, and the accurate interpretation and communication of medical information becomes a literal *Tower of Babel*.

Although nurses not certified in medical interpretation or translation should not adopt the role of official interpreter for patients who do not speak English, nurses do indeed have a responsibility—morally, ethically, and professionally—to assist patients in understanding the trajectory of their care. This may include enlisting other professionals who can fill gaps in communication and culture that may stand in the way of understanding—and ultimately, patient outcomes.

Nurses Are Cultural Ombudspeople

As the frequent conduit between physicians, patients, families, and the rest of the healthcare delivery team, nurses must finesse the nuances of diagnosis, treatment, and patient education in a manner that honors the needs, beliefs, and cultural practices of the patient while also adhering to the most central aspects of the treatment plan. Nurses play a key role in this dance of language, education, and medical intervention, and the elicitation of patient "buy-in" largely rests on the shoulders of the nurse as he or she navigates the shifting waters of culture, medicine, and nursing.

Ascertaining a patient's beliefs and cultural norms can be a time-consuming business when a nurse is hard pressed to care for his or her many patients. Although time may seem like a precious commodity for the busy nurse, we must also consider the precious commodity of the patient's belief system and values, seeking ways to bridge the gaps that can potentially throw a wrench in the treatment plan.

For instance, one patient's religious beliefs may preclude receiving blood transfusions, whereas another patient may refuse antibiotics or a medication derived from animals. In these cases, the earnest nurse must not allow his or her own judgments about the patient's beliefs and values to poison the nurse–patient relationship, and it is a skilled nurse indeed who can rise above his or her own judgments to meet patients in their world.

A Tapestry of Collaboration

The nurse, through skillful and compassionate communication, may succeed in bridging divides that could otherwise thwart the most comprehensive treatment plan. It is through the art of listening, speaking authentically and clearly, and honoring the

Continued

Confident Voices—cont'd

beliefs and values of the patient that the nurse knits together a tapestry of collaboration that can successfully deliver the positive outcomes that the entire team—and the patient and family—ultimately desire.

Biography

Keith Carlson has been a nurse since 1996. He is the well-known blogger behind the award-winning blog Digital Doorway (digitaldoorway.blogspot.com) and a widely read freelance nurse writer. He is also the cohost of RNFM Radio (rnfmradio.com), a popular Internet radio station devoted to the nursing profession. As a Board Certified Nurse Coach working under the auspices of Nurse Keith Coaching (nursekeith.com), Carlson's passion is helping nurses and healthcare professionals create ultimate satisfaction in both their personal and professional lives.

CULTURAL COMPETENCE

The formal term for accepting diversity in professional practice is **cultural competence**. Cultural competence is necessary for nurses to work collaboratively within a diverse workforce and provide patient-centered care to *all* people. Whereas patient-centered care identifies, respects, and addresses differences in patients' values, preferences, and expressed needs (National Research Council, 2003), cultural competence is defined as "[a] set of integrated attitudes, knowledge and skills that enable a health care professional or organization to care effectively for patients from diverse cultures, groups and communities" (Gilbert, 2003, p. 11).

One of the most important concepts that students need to understand in order to develop cultural competence is **dominant culture**, which is the established or majority culture of any group, community, or organization. The dominant culture drives the assumptions that people in an environment make regarding language, religion, behavior, values, rituals, and social customs. Similar to implicit rules in an organizational culture, dominant culture can be very powerful in setting expectations and governing behavior, and it can be intentionally or unintentionally oppressive to those who are not part of the culture. Nurses must consider what it feels like to be a member of a nondominant culture in order to eliminate presumptions or exclusionary behavior. One way to develop empathy for being a minority member in a dominant culture is to envision how it might feel to be in any of the following situations:

- A nurse in a meeting with a group of physicians
- A male nursing student in a class of women
- A homosexual nurse in a department made up of heterosexual colleagues
- A Hispanic nursing student as part of an otherwise Caucasian unit

Each of these instances is intended to inspire a sense of what it might feel like to be different from the majority. In a dominant culture, prejudices related to how someone dresses, speaks, or dates are common, even when no judgments are expressed or overtly visible. The need for affiliation and for love or acceptance, part of Maslow's hierarchy (1999), may feel threatened in a culture in which all signs suggest that one does not belong.

Cultural imposition and *cultural sensitivity* are two concepts that provide additional insight into the development of cultural competency: "Cultural imposition intrusively applies the majority cultural view to individuals and families. Prescribing a special diet without regard to the client's culture and limiting visitors to immediate family borders is cultural imposition. In this context, healthcare providers must be careful in expressing their cultural values too strongly until cultural issues are more fully understood.... Cultural sensitivity is experienced when neutral language—both verbal and nonverbal—is used in a way that reflects sensitivity and appreciation for the diversity of another. It is conveyed when words, phrases, categorizations, etc., are intentionally avoided, especially when referring to any individual who may interpret them as impolite or offensive" (Giger et al., 2007, p. 96).

Effective communication skills and a foundation of emotional awareness form an extremely valuable basis for developing cultural competence. A nurse's awareness of self and others' needs, beliefs, and desires, as well as his or her willingness to reflect on and challenge assumptions, show ownership for limitations, validate different perspectives, and develop genuine curiosity, are rooted in this skill set. Consequently, nurses who are respectful communicators will be better prepared to be collaborative partners in diverse teams. When nurses are part of the majority population, emotional intelligence, curiosity, and perspective taking will be essential for honoring minority colleagues and patients; at the other end of the spectrum, assertiveness has a heightened role for minority nurses who must express their voices in dominant cultures.

The AACN's (2008) *Tool Kit of Resources for Cultural Competent Education for Baccalaureate Nurses* lists attributes that reflect cultural competence in clinical practice:

- "Awareness of personal culture, values, beliefs, and behaviors.
- Knowledge of and respect for different cultures.
- Skills in interacting and responding to individuals from other cultures.
- Acknowledgement about importance of culture and incorporation at all levels.
- Assessment of cross-cultural relations.
- Vigilance toward the dynamics that result from cultural differences expansion of cultural knowledge.
- Adaptation of services to meet culturally unique needs." (p. 13)

In day-to-day practice, nurses will have many opportunities to develop cultural competence. Nurses should try to use inviting language to integrate clinical expertise with development and application of cultural competency (e.g., "I'm wondering how the cost of medication to control your blood pressure might affect your ability to pay rent or buy groceries." or "Help me understand your family's beliefs about death and dying.").

BEING OPEN TO DIVERSITY AND CREATING A CLIMATE OF INCLUSION

When fear and judgment are absent, diversity can lead to occasions of cooperative creativity, learning, and productive conflict. Yet creating such opportunities is not so simple. Nurses are human and are subject to prejudices, insecurities, and fears about people and things different from them just like anyone else might be. Feelings of superiority or inferiority, judgments about religious beliefs or sexual activity, and racial bias may have roots in profound core life experiences. Growing up in a family with a rigid religious doctrine, surviving a rape or molestation, and losing a loved one to gun violence are examples of experiences that could understandably contribute to fear, closed-mindedness, or generalizations toward groups of people with which

Consultant Commentary

My first year out of nursing school, I cared for a 16-year-old Caucasian patient who had shot herself in the abdomen with her father's handgun because she thought she was preg- nant. She was extremely worried that her father would be angry, not only that she had been sexually active, but also with an older Japanese man because her father was a World War II veteran with a history of violence and bigotry. The young woman's emotional fear was so powerful that taking her own life seemed like a better option than revealing her relationship or pregnancy.

It turned out she wasn't pregnant, but she ended up paralyzed from the waist down as a result of her injuries. As a young and inexperienced nurse, I was shocked. I found it hard to understand why her parents would create such a fearful environment or why she would be compelled to take such a drastic and irreversible measure. Even 25 years later, as I write this, it brings up powerful feelings for me. Would her father have shunned an unwed pregnant daughter? Where did his fears and bigotry come from? Did he feel his identity and survival threatened? Could her mother have supported her, or was she, too, afraid? I may not have all the answers to these questions, but I think in asking them, I make room for compassion—for the young woman, the man she was involved with, and her parents.

Another tricky, although less emotionally charged, issue I faced more recently in my career came in working with a young African American man from Nigeria. He was a certi- fied nurse assistant working on a dementia unit where all the residents were white. His skin was deeply black, his accent thick, and his English imperfect. As he gently took patients' hands to help them stand, he would say, "Come on, Mama, you can do it." I was unsure if this was inappropriate because I mostly avoid using terms of endearment such as "honey" or "dear" with patients for fear of seeming patronizing and condescending. How- ever, in talking with this nurse assistant, I learned that in his culture, the elderly are held in high regard and, in turn, are frequently called "mama" and "papa." I could tell patients felt safe with him and that he clearly displayed respect and dignity for them nonverbally.

Although the instances are very different, they forced me to really consider what it's like for those who are a minority in a dominant culture and to reflect on how I interact with them, whether they are a patient or a colleague.

an individual might associate these experiences. Nurses who find themselves emotionally unable to deal with certain types of people should get professional support from a psychologist or counselor to help sort through painful feelings and develop healthy coping mechanisms. Nev- ertheless, given that nurses may work in diverse teams and must provide care for people from all walks of life, it is essential for nurses to have awareness about any limitations. After these limits are acknowledged, nurses must be vigilant to not compromise care for any patients who are part of a population that they have a bias toward and must be able to set aside fears or judg- ments. It is also important for nurses to honor their own emotional safety; with or without pro- fessional support, this can be tough to balance. Ideally, nurses will find a way to champion a strong and compassionate stance around diversity and will learn to step back when they cannot.

Beyond just being open to diversity, nurses must learn to create a **climate of inclusion**. This can be accomplished by a few different strategies. First is through the use of inclusive language, which was touched on earlier in the discussion about cultural sensitivity. This might mean say- ing "Happy Holidays" instead of or in addition to "Merry Christmas." In a healthcare setting with a dominant Christian culture, nurses could take it a step further by asking, "Do you cele-brate anything special in your culture this time of year?" Assuming someone doesn't celebrate a dominant culture's holiday may be a presumption, but when aligned with true curiosity, it is likely to be appreciated even if wrong. Another time to use inclusive language is when asking a colleague or patient about their personal relationships. Nurses should be careful with terms such as "boyfriend" or "girlfriend" and "husband" or "wife" because they are inadvertently ex-clusive in a heterosexual-dominant culture. Simply asking if the person is "dating someone" demonstrates openness to whatever gender that "someone" may be. Members of dominant cultures who find it inconvenient to make extra efforts like these should be encouraged to reflect on their own attitudes about diversity.

A second strategy in becoming intentionally inclusive is to work on a committee or project with members of a minority. This may happen naturally in the course of working together, but leaders also can create such opportunities, and individuals can seek them out. Collaborating on a committee or workshop creates a basis of common experience and a chance to learn about each other as individuals. This strategy builds trust and positive relationships while diminishing exclusion. As a result, the positive elements of diversity can thrive.

The third strategy is to incorporate a philosophy of "no innocent bystanders" into interper-sonal dynamics. The concept originated in educational settings in an effort to create safe learn-ing environments and eliminate bullying behaviors (Cohen, 2001). Nurses can use the philosophy by speaking up when inappropriate behavior is occurring, such as gossiping about someone's religion or telling a joke about a minority (e.g., "I think it is inappropriate to tell jokes about Muslims" or "Please stop gossiping about the new nurse's learning disability"). Nurse leaders take on responsibility in ensuring an inclusive environment. For example, senior organizational leaders can help by creating, role-modeling, and enforcing a policy that holds all parties accountable for speaking up when inappropriate behaviors are witnessed. Such in-terventions will help counteract a toxic dominant culture in which bullying or discrimination may be tacitly condoned. Managers and charge nurses can help by not laughing at inappropriate jokes, participating in any inappropriate behavior, and reminding staff to be professional.

Inclusion should not only be practiced by nurses but also encouraged by nurses in others. Occasionally, patients refuse care provided by the opposite sex or by someone from a particular ethnic group. Although some organizations may honor such patient preferences, it is important for organizations also to consider how such requests may place a burden on select staff. Nurses can aid patients in being inclusive by listening to their concerns and making sure to validate them (e.g., "It sounds like you would not feel comfortable having a man give you a shower. Can you share more about your worries?" or "Is there some way we could help you feel more comfortable interacting with our diverse workforce? Maybe if you had a chance to meet some of them first?"). Certainly, a patient who has religious beliefs that forbid exposure to the oppo-site sex or has experienced a traumatic event associated with a person of a particular race does not need to be pushed or further traumatized unnecessarily. Yet the bigger goal of helping people become more inclusive may be reached from such a conversation and subsequent experiences. Even when patients insist on limiting their caregivers, such a conversation will introduce an alternative way of thinking and may inspire reflection and growth.

RANKISM AND DIGNITY

Another interesting lens through which to consider the importance of respectful relationships that encompass diversity is **rankism**. In his book, *Somebodies and Nobodies: Overcoming the*

Abuse of Rank, philosopher and physicist Robert Fuller (2004) explains that "[r]acism, sexism, anti-Semitism, ageism, and others all depend on their existence on differences of social rank that in turn reflect underlying power differences, so they are forms of rankism" (p. 2). He goes on to portray how destructive rankism is: "Rankism erodes the will to learn, distorts personal relationships, taxes economic productivity, and stokes ethnic hatred. It is the cause of dysfunctionality, and sometimes even violence, in families, schools and the workplace" (p. 3). In a 2011 TED talk, Fuller provides this concise definition: "Rankism is a degrading assertion of power or rank" (Fuller, 2011, 10:25).

Abuse of power is present within many healthcare systems and other environments in which nurses serve. Fuller's work is especially helpful in identifying insidious power advantages found in dominant cultures, such as a toxic hierarchy, or discriminatory practices by those in positional or high-status power. Examples of rankism in healthcare include a surgeon who humiliates a member of the operating room team for making a simple mistake or a group of nurses who exclude one nurse for petty reasons.

Fuller's (2011) solution for fighting the pervasiveness of rankism is through promoting dignity. Dignity calls on every person to recognize an equal and inherent worth in all people and to remember that having expertise, money, or positional power does not give permission for someone to assume more importance than others. A nurse who treats all others with dignity will always be prepared to deal with the diversity she sees every day. Ultimately, treating others with dignity is an attitude, whereas respectful communication is the mechanism for conveying it.

Confident Voices

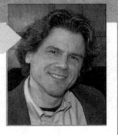

Paul Gross, MD
Assistant Professor

We're Not So Very Different

Beneath our uniforms or gowns, you and I—clinician and patient, nurse and doctor—are not so very different from one another. Appreciating this reality, and acting on it, can make all the difference.

A healthcare professional who sees himself or herself as a potential patient will likely adopt a more empathetic approach toward a sick person. And a patient's appreciation of a health professional's humanity helps to create a connection powerful enough to relieve distress and promote healing.

From personal experience, I can also say that cutting through barriers and forming a bond with a patient is, for me, *the* most rewarding part of my profession.

How curious, then, that our similarities are rarely emphasized in medical training. In fact, it's just the opposite.

From the earliest days of my medical education, there was something about the way in which patients were presented to us—in the form of corpses, diseased anatomy specimens, or stained tissues under the microscope—that made them seem like a different species. They were old. They were sick. In fact, they were usually dead.

Confident Voices—cont'd

Even when live patients were paraded before us for purposes of display and questioning, there was something about the process that made them seem other-worldly. They were diseased. They'd abused themselves. Implicitly, they weren't as smart as we were.

Not surprisingly, my fellow students and I, faced with these unfortunate specters of old age, illness, and death, often assumed an us-versus-them attitude. It was tempting to believe—we all fervently *wanted* to believe—that we could outwit and escape their fate.

At the same time, our teachers realized that we needed to learn to talk to patients, so my classmates and I dutifully learned certain principles of communication. We were taught to elicit patients' concerns, ask open-ended questions, and listen non-judgmentally to their responses. We were told to look patients in the eye and to as-sume an attitude of empathetic understanding. These tools of communication made sense—and they often worked.

And, yet, I couldn't help but notice how rarely these powerful tools were used by our teachers in their dealings with us. How often did someone in authority ask me, "How are you doing?" How often were we encouraged to tell the truth about our learning experience? How often did our instructors hear us out, listen nonjudgmen-tally, and then act to address the stresses or indignities we were enduring?

Implicit in the difference between the way we were supposed to treat patients and the way that we ourselves were treated was that we students were somehow different from our patients. We didn't need kid-glove treatment because *their* vulnerabilities were not *our* vulnerabilities.

And what about members of our healthcare team—nurses, let's say? What were we taught about them?

Remarkably little. Which is to say, little educational time that I can remember was spent reflecting on the role of a nurse or the duties of a nurse. And *no* time was spent reflecting on communication between physicians and nurses. (Although I can recall a fair amount of informal griping during residency about how certain nurses on certain floors treated us. And a wiser senior resident would counsel the impulsive intern to be polite and respectful—because an irate nurse could make your life miserable.)

The lack of instruction devoted to the nurse's role and to communication between doctor and nurse carried two implied falsehoods: first, that whatever nurses did was not critical to the health of patients; and second, that we and they were also some-how different.

Continued

Confident Voices—cont'd

It was in part to address these artificial barriers that exist among physicians, our patients, and fellow health professionals that, a half-dozen years ago, several colleagues and I launched an online publication called *Pulse—Voices From the Heart of Medicine* (pulsevoices.org). Our goal was to create a common space where we could all gather, sharing what it's like to be our vulnerable selves, in our various roles, confronting moments of illness.

Every Friday, *Pulse* subscribers receive by e-mail a first-person story or poem about healthcare, written by a patient or doctor, a nurse or caregiver, another health professional, or a family member. One such story, "Nineteen Steps" (pulsevoices.org/archive/stories/279-nineteen-steps) by nurse Priscilla Mainardi, recounts with humor and poignancy her efforts to balance her job's conflicting tugs: the many concrete tasks she must accomplish on the one hand, and a tearful, dying patient who needs her listening ear on the other.

These stories and poems serve to remind us that, fundamentally, we're not so different. And *Pulse*'s readers have responded approvingly—because that's something we all long to hear. We want to know that our doctor aches just like us, that our nurse is smart and sensitive to our needs, and that our patient notices the difference between care that is unfeeling and care that is humane, just as we do.

One wonders how the delivery of healthcare might change if health professionals remembered our similarities when dealing with our patients or speaking with our healthcare colleagues. And what would the collaboration between nurses and doctors look like if we could see one another not as different creatures, wearing uniforms that symbolize our differences, but rather as alternate incarnations of ourselves?

Biography

In addition to serving as president of *Pulse—Voices From the Heart of Medicine*, Paul Gross, MD, is assistant professor in the Department of Family and Social Medicine at Albert Einstein College of Medicine/Montefiore Medical Center, where he teaches narrative medicine to residents. His stories about medical practice and family life have appeared in *American Family Physician*, *Journal of Family Practice*, *Hippocrates*, *The Sun*, *Diversions*, and *Town & Country*. He also conducts award-winning writing workshops for medical professionals.

CASE STUDY

James is an RN who teaches both classroom and clinical courses in an Associate Degree Nursing program. The program is offered in a community that is primarily white, including James. There are 24 students in his "Introduction to Nursing" class. James's class is made up of five African American students, two male and three female. There are two Asian women in the class, and one Hispanic female. The rest of the class is Caucasian, all females with the exception of one male. In today's class, James shares a personal story about how an older female patient once refused his assistance because of his gender. This sparks an increasingly animated conversation in which some of the men and non-Caucasian women in the class describe different instances in their nursing experience thus far when they felt they were the victim of someone's prejudices. Out of the corner of his eye, James notices a young, white female student in the back corner roll her eyes and mutter something to herself. He decides not to make an issue of it in class, but later wonders if he missed an important teaching opportunity.

Discussion Questions

1. What known dominant and minority cultures exist in this classroom? What are some ways that members of the dominant cultures might exhibit cultural imposition during class? What opportunities exist for members of the dominant cultures to demonstrate cultural sensitivity?
2. What other cultures might exist that are not obvious in the description?
3. With respect to the material in this chapter, what concerns do you think James might have about the student who rolled her eyes? About the students who shared their experiences with prejudice?
4. How could James have responded to the situation in a way that would have encouraged inclusion and helped the students develop culture competence?

SUMMARY

Working with diverse populations requires an openness to learn about different ways of being, from the food someone eats to philosophies on life and death and from musical traditions to alternative family compositions. A nurse's ability to be inclusive of all types of people can be limited by fears, assumptions, or judgments that human beings are prone to when they feel inferior or superior to others or threatened in some way. Respectful communication, sensitivity to others, and a willingness to treat others with dignity are essential for creating and sustaining environments that are safe for everyone.

Reflection Questions

1. Think of a situation at work or in school in which you are a member of a dominant culture. Do you feel any sense of superiority in relationship to minority members you are working or in school with? Explain or write about your feelings. What could you do ensure that minority members feel welcome and safe to fully participate in work or school activities?

2. Think of a situation at work or in school in which you are a member of a minority culture. Do you feel any sense of inferiority in relationship to members of the dominant culture? Explain or write about your feelings. What might help you feel safe and welcome to ensure that you fully participate in work or school activities?

3. Should members of the minority cultures be held to the same degree of responsibility regarding creating inclusive cultures? Support your reasoning.

References

American Association of Colleges of Nursing. (2008). *Tool kit of resources for cultural competent education for baccalaureate nurses.* Retrieved from www.aacn.nche.edu/education-resources/toolkit.pdf

Budden, J. S., Zhong, E. H., Moulton, P., & Cimiotti, J. P. (2013) Supplement: The National Council of State Boards of Nursing and the Forum of State Nursing Workforce Centers 2013 national workforce survey of registered nurses. *Journal of Nursing Regulation, 4*(2), S1–S72.

Cohen, J. (Ed.). (2001). *Caring classrooms/intelligent schools: The social emotional education of young children.* New York: Teachers College Press.

Fang, D., Li, Y., Arietti, R., & Bednash, G. D. (2014a). *2013–2014 Enrollment and graduations in baccalaureate and graduate programs in nursing.* Washington, DC: American Association of Colleges of Nursing.

Fang, D., Li, Y., Arietti, R., & Bednash, G. D. (2014b). *2013–2014 Salaries of instructional and administrative nursing faculty in baccalaureate and graduate programs in nursing.* Washington, DC: American Association of Colleges of Nursing.

Fuller, R. W. (2004). *Somebodies and nobodies: Overcoming the abuse of rank.* British Columbia, Canada: New Society Publishers.

Fuller, R. W. (2011, March 23). TedxBerkeley—Robert Fuller—Rankism. Retrieved from www.youtube.com/watch?v=djM6cZb8kak

Giger, J., Davidhizar, R. E., Purnell, L., Harden, J. T., Phillips, J., & Strickland, O. (2007). American Academy of Nursing Expert Panel Report: Developing cultural competence to eliminate health disparities in ethnic minorities and other vulnerable populations. *Journal of Transcultural Nursing, 18*(2), 95–102.

Gilbert, J. M. (Ed.). (2003). *Principles and recommended standards for cultural competence education of health care professionals.* Woodland, CA: California Endowment. Retrieved from www.calendow.org/uploadedFiles/principles_standards_cultural_competence.pdf

Maslow, A. (1999). *Toward a psychology of being* (3rd ed.). New York: Wiley & Sons. (Original work published 1986).

National Research Council. (2003). *Health professions education: A bridge to quality.* Washington, DC: National Academies Press.

U.S. Census Bureau. (2012). U.S. Census Bureau projections show a slower growing, older, more diverse nation a half century from now. Retrieved from www.census.gov/newsroom/releases/archives/population/cb12-243.html

Williams, S. D., Hansen, K., Wright, K. F., Burnley, J., Koyama, K., Smithey, M., ... White, K. M. (2014). Nursing in 3D: Workforce diversity, health disparities, social determinants of health. *Public Health Reports, 129*(Suppl. 2).

CHAPTER 14

Health Information Technology and Digital Communication

LEARNING OBJECTIVES

- Discuss the importance of communication and interpersonal relationships in implementation of health information technology systems
- Identify how assertiveness and listening can eliminate workarounds
- Explain differences between face-to-face and digital communication
- Describe privacy concerns and appropriate use of digital communication

KEY TERMS

- Health information technology
- Electronic medical record
- Bar code medication administration
- Workaround
- Telenursing

Health information technology and social media have introduced new ways of communicating in healthcare systems and the nursing practice. Although not intended to be a comprehensive evaluation of any specific health information technology, this chapter provides insight into the critical value of respectful communication in the advancement and use of any technology related to patient care. In addition, students will explore personal and professional responsibilities associated with digital communication, including e-mail and social media.

HEALTH INFORMATION TECHNOLOGY

The advancing technology in healthcare provides access to huge volumes of rapidly evolving information, offering the possibility of safer, more informed, and streamlined care. This **health information technology** also brings challenges in terms of implementation, standardization, utilization, and patient safety. Fundamental communication skills are related to the success or failure of any health information technology system. Electronic medical records and barcoded medication administration are two important systems nurses will use that illustrate these points.

Electronic Medical Records

An **electronic medical record** (EMR) is the digital equivalent of the traditional paper chart and contains a patient's medical history from a particular hospital, outpatient, or home health facility, with sections for nurses' notes, doctors' orders, laboratory results, radiology reports, physical therapy instructions, code status, and other pertinent information. Like paper charts, EMRs are maintained by the facility so that information from previous visits or hospitalizations is available to clinicians. EMRs are one part of a larger set of electronic records that includes electronic health records, personal health records, and computerized provider order entry systems. There is some overlapping of terms among these records; a useful glossary can be found at HealthIT.gov (www.healthit.gov/policy-researchers-implementers/glossary), along with many other related resources.

Potential benefits of EMRs include better tracking of patient information over time, such as trends in weight or blood pressure, and easy identification of a patient's need for screening or prevention measures. However, there have been barriers associated with implementing EMRs. Albert Boonstra and Manda Broekhuis (2010) found eight main categories of barriers: financial, technical, time, psychological, social, legal, organizational, and change process. Concerns have also emerged about patient safety stemming from poor human–computer interactions or loss of data, such as dosing errors, failure to detect fatal illnesses, and delayed treatment (Institute of Medicine [IOM], 2012). The IOM report *Health IT and Patient Safety: Building Safer Systems for Better Care* (IOM, 2012) details how the evolution of health information technology has been plagued with problems despite the promises that it holds in making healthcare safer. One of the most important points made in the IOM report is that "[s]afety is an emergent property of a larger system that takes into account not just the software but also how it is used by clinicians" (p. 3). In other words, there must be awareness of the role that communication and interpersonal relationships have in how technology such as EMR is used by clinicians.

The importance of communication and human relationships in the implementation of technology was evident at the onset of EMR. The first commercial EMR was the Technicon Medical Information System, designed by Lockheed engineers and implemented at El Camino Hospital in central California (Buchanan, 1984). Neilson Buchanan wrote an experiential paper describing the collaborative process between the developers at Lockheed and the users at El Camino, which took place in several stages and over a period of almost 20 years, beginning in the mid-1960s. Perhaps more widely recognized in retrospect, the subtle cooperative spirit that was present throughout the process was likely integral to the successful implementation and evolution of the system. That healthy communication and interpersonal relationships existed throughout the process is obvious throughout Buchanan's paper. For instance, because the nurses were teaching the program to the physicians, one can surmise that the doctors listened respectfully to the nurses' expertise. Likewise, because the nurses were the ones chosen to learn the program initially, one can infer that they were generally respected in the organization and engaged in the initiative.

From Buchanan's observations of the development of EMR, certain lessons can be applied in the implementation of any health information technology: Stakeholders must be engaged in the design and implementation of the system; there must be opportunities for quick and meaningful feedback loops when problems occur or new ideas are generated; and team members must share information, help each other problem-solve, and manage conflict productively. If these guidelines are adhered to, then the likelihood of successful use of the technology is much greater.

An interesting historical perspective comes from Dr. Linda Thede (2012). In her article, "Informatics: Where Is It?" she depicts a time in the early 1980s when new technology was offering great promise: "We envisioned such things as minimal time spent in documentation, working together with patients to document past history and care received, a lifetime healthcare record, and the use of aggregated data to improve nursing practice. Informatics, we believed, would free nurses and other healthcare professionals to spend more time with patients and minimize the pain of documentation" (para. 4). She points out that progress toward this vision has been made since then, including an increase in organizations' use of health information technology in clinical departments, development of informatics courses and a career path for nurses, and the Centers for Medicare and Medicaid Services' (2014) "Meaningful Use" program, which offers a financial incentive for using EMRs to collect data that will improve patient care. Thede also reports on areas that have been problematic, such as poor screen design, lack of system integration, failure to implement informatics principles, and an inability for systems to share data with other departments. With roughly 30 years in related work, Thede (2012) concludes that "[o]ne thing that we early dreamers failed to consider was the cultural changes that would be needed to reach our dreams. One of the biggest of these needs is a move from a silo mentality to a multidisciplinary perspective" (para. 13). This move can easily be reframed into creating a collaborative culture with a basis of respectful communication that fosters the intended use of technology in delivering safe, quality care.

Consider what might take place in a hospital without a collaborative culture attempting to integrate an EMR. For instance, a nurse who has been humiliated by a physician during a conversation about a patient might understandably avoid unnecessary contact with this physician if he is on the unit. This nurse may be well versed in the computer system, but what is the likelihood that she will teach the doctor how to use it or that the doctor would be open to learning from the nurse? Consciously or unconsciously, direct or indirect, the impact that frontline users of a system have on its success or failure is significant. Healthcare professionals must appreciate how destructive toxic relationships and lack of respectful communication can be in implementing any new change, let alone a complex, system-wide change like EMR.

Ann Farrell, an emergency room nurse at El Camino Hospital during the EMR implementation and currently a health information technology consultant, reflects on the experience in Thede's article: "The collaborative culture and respect for the role of RNs was reflected in system design. MIS [management information systems] provided more functionality and better integration for nurses than we see in most systems today; requirements of the healthcare providers drove the technical innovations" (quoted in Thede, 2012, para. 3). This raises an alarming question: What is driving technical innovations today? The answer is beyond the scope of this text and is likely a combination of influences such as profit making, budgetary constraints, patient safety, and legal and regulatory influences. The compelling take-home message for students is that the individual and collective voices of nurses at all levels should have major influence on the development of technology associated with patient care. In order for that to become a reality, nurses must practice respectful communication, collaborate effectively, and contribute to healthy workplace cultures.

Bar-Code Medication Administration

Bar-code medication administration (BCMA) provides another opportunity to explore the case for effective communication, positive work relationships, and a healthy culture as a foundation for enhancing outcomes associated with health information technology. A BCMA system "utilizes bar-coded medication doses, patient identification bracelets, and nurse staff badges

Confident Voices

Brittney Wilson, BSN, RN
Clinical Informatics Nurse and Professional Blogger

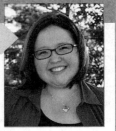

Avoiding Potential Pitfalls With Electronic Medical Records and Social Media

In recent years, technology has changed healthcare in so many ways. It is hard to pinpoint a single area of healthcare and nursing that hasn't been made better by technology. But unfortunately, the rapid adaptation of digital communication has left room for error. With use of electronic medical records (EMRs) and social media specifically, there are potential pitfalls that nurses and other healthcare workers need to be aware of.

One of the biggest pitfalls that a nurse can make when using an EMR is overdocumenting. Long gone are the days of the wordy narrative notes. These have been replaced with concise checkboxes and dropdown menus; yet some nurses still feel the need to write elaborate narratives detailing every aspect of a patient's care. This can cause many issues for nurses, including wasted time and potential legal liabilities. There is no need to document care twice, and in doing so nurses might alter details and create inconsistencies in documentation, which could create a potential issue if they were ever called to defend the care they delivered. Another thing to consider about excessive narrative notes is that these data cannot be captured and reported on. In order to meet meaningful use requirements and to create data that are useful to improve patient care, discrete data (gathered through checkboxes, dropdown menus, or other fields with predefined answers) must be recorded.

With smartphones in hand, nurses and healthcare workers can express their thoughts and opinions whenever they get the urge. This can be a potential pitfall if they are not clear on social media etiquette and HIPAA guidelines. Every nurse should read his or her hospital's policy regarding social media as well as the American Nurses Association guidelines on social media use (www.nursingworld .org/FunctionalMenuCategories/AboutANA/Social-Media). In addition, nurses must make sure they are explicitly clear on what is and isn't appropriate on social media. The three pieces of advice on social media that will save nurses the most grief are as follows:

1. Don't say anything on social media that you wouldn't say in front of your boss or your human resources manager.
2. Don't identify your employer on your social media profiles, and don't post to social media while you are on the clock.
3. Be respectful of the patients you serve, and don't violate their privacy or respect by posting identifying information online.

Confident Voices—cont'd

Social media is a new form of communication that sometimes gets misused, but more often it's simply misunderstood. Look at social media as an opportunity to expand your professional network and build additional pathways for collaboration.

As a technology and social media enthusiast, I am beyond thrilled with all the improvements technology has made to patient care. I also see the impact that social media is making on healthcare now and will continue to make in the years to come. It is up to nurses and other healthcare workers to ensure that we use the tools that we are given wisely. These technologies are extremely powerful, and with great power comes great responsibility.

Biography

Brittney Wilson, RN, BSN, is a clinical informatics nurse practicing in Atlanta, Georgia. In her day job, she gets to do what she loves every day: combine technology and healthcare to improve patient outcomes. Wilson is the author of *The Nerdy Nurse's Guide to Technology* (2014, Sigma Theta Tau International). She is a social media influencer and blogs about nursing, technology, healthcare, parenting, and various lifestyle topics at TheNerdyNurse.com. You can also connect with her on twitter (@TheNerdyNurse) or Facebook (www.facebook.com/TheNerdyNurse).

to facilitate the *five rights* (right patient, right medication, right dose, right time and right route) of medication administration. The BCMA system includes a server and a wireless handheld device (or a tethered device) coupled with software that interfaces with a hospital's information system. The system is often integrated with a patient unit-based automatic dispensing machine (ADM) and a pharmacy packaging and dispensing robot" (Gooder, 2011, para. 7).

BCMA represents another advancement in health information technology that offers significant hope in reducing medication errors associated with dispensing and transcription. Research has shown "that BCMA technology can reduce medication errors from 65% to 86%" (Pennsylvania Patient Safety Authority, 2008, para. 3). Yet studies also point to concerns about nursing attitudes, such as satisfaction or frustration (Gooder, 2011), and a high frequency of workarounds or shortcuts (discussed later in this section) involving the use of BCMA systems (Koppel, Wetterneck, Telles, & Karsh, 2008). Valerie Gooder (2011) found that nurses' satisfaction decreased with the use of BCMA systems and concluded that "[b]efore any decisions are made regarding the overall effectiveness of BCMA, hospitals first need to determine whether the benefits are negated by nurses' resistance to the change and how that resistance can be minimized" (para. 41).

Nurses' resistance to change, wherever it might come from, certainly can influence the use of BCMA and any other health information technology. Resistance can run the gamut from not fully embracing change to shutting down and not contributing ideas, and from not doing everything possible to make a new program work to seeking out and exploiting negative consequences that might arise. Nurses who are resistant may align with colleagues who feel similarly and consequently develop informal but destructive power. Resistance can be fueled by organizations that promote leaders who don't invite and listen to input from staff, who assume that staff have little of value to add, or who believe that it doesn't matter how staff are affected by change. As mentioned previously, for a system to be implemented successfully, there must be respectful communication among stakeholders. This does not mean that that every nurse has to have input into every new system, or that leaders should spend all of their time listening to suggestions from nurses, but at the bare minimum, a culture in which giving and receiving constructive feedback are valued must be in place.

Workarounds

Health information technology systems like EMR and BCMA affect the workflow of all nurses. When staff members have problems with new equipment but have no channels for having those issues addressed in an effective or timely manner, they are likely to develop a **workaround**. A workaround is an alternative process that does not follow protocols or policies; it may save time, be easier, and allow completion of necessary tasks when support is not available to do them properly. Workarounds are frequently used when technology interferes with workflow, requires more time to use it, or seems to cause more problems than it solves. Students may see workarounds used in clinical rotations when nurses skip steps or modify processes such as BCMA. However, in the end, workarounds undermine the safe practices that the technology is intended to ensure.

Ross Koppel and colleagues (2008) observed and shadowed nurses using BCMA systems at five hospitals. The authors identified 15 types of workarounds, including affixing patient identification bar codes to computer carts, scanners, doorjambs, or nurses' belt rings, and carrying several patients' prescanned medications on carts (pp. 418–419). The authors identified 31 causes of workarounds, such as unreadable medication bar codes (e.g., crinkled, smudged, torn, missing, covered by another label), malfunctioning scanners, unreadable or missing patient identification wristbands (e.g., chewed, soaked, missing), non–bar-coded medications, failing batteries, and uncertain wireless connectivity (pp. 418–421).

Although workarounds are not generally practiced or talked about openly, because they are breaking protocol, they may become habitual. The links between workarounds with health information technology systems to underlying communication, collaboration, and organizational culture issues are not necessarily obvious. Ongoing and timely feedback loops must be cultivated in the design, implementation, and quality improvement processes (e.g., in the case of BCMA, ensuring that batteries are readily available or instituting an easy process for replacing or checking on patient identification wristbands). A feedback loop that is either too long or laborious to complete often results in workarounds, whereas a feedback loop that is timely and collaborative can lead to solutions and demonstrate a collaborative process with end users.

Consultant Commentary

From the perspective of teaching communication topics, advancing technology has provided me many challenges and opportunities. When teaching a behavioral approach to communication, being in the room with students is very valuable. When face-to-face with students, I can pick up on emotional cues that might signal eagerness, hesitancy, or even resistance to participate; pick up on tension that exists between students; and observe what kind of informal power hierarchy exists within the group. In the room, in the moment, there are rich opportunities for individuals and teams to learn to work more collaboratively together.

Consultant Commentary—cont'd

On the other hand, there is great value in technology for teaching communication. Videos on YouTube are wonderful resources that I have referenced several times in this book. I also worked with my colleagues, Stephanie Frederick and Judy White, as well as six other experts from all over the United States, to record a Google Hangout that introduces and demonstrates new ideas about medical improv. Yes, there were many headaches (e.g., making sure the participants knew how to use their computer cameras and microphones, integrating PowerPoint presentations into the live event, making sure we all knew how to use the Google interface and related apps), and we had glitches. But we did eventually succeed!

I am now getting ready to pilot a project with American Healthcare Media to do webinars on communication-related topics. American Healthcare Media is experimenting with new webcam technology as a way to offer continuing education. Each episode will be live and recorded. This will allow for the exchange of perspectives, role-modeling of difficult conversations, and education on the topic itself. Most important, we will reach a much bigger audience than we could have by offering the same thing in an in-person forum.

Ultimately, whether in a healthcare or teaching setting, technology used wisely can provide great benefits as an alternative to human interface.

DIGITAL COMMUNICATION

Just as health information technology systems such as EMR and BCMA are changing the face of the healthcare industry, so is digital communication. With the integration of smartphones and tablets into the healthcare setting, staff members are now expected to text, e-mail, video chat, and use social media as part of their jobs. This section is not meant to fully cover digital communication, but rather to illuminate considerations and interpersonal dynamics that are associated with it, whether nurses are using digital communication to reach patients in other locations or as a tool in the traditional healthcare setting.

Telenursing

Nurses now routinely perform parts of their job on the phone or through e-mailing, texting, and live video streaming—all part of what is now called **telenursing**. Telenursing is any nursing practice that takes place over the phone, through electronic communication such as e-mail and text, and through any virtual medium that provides live video streaming. When practicing telenursing, nurses must be careful to follow practice guidelines and triage or case management protocols for identifying and assessing patients as well as providing any nursing advice. As with providing care in a traditional healthcare setting, clarifying and validating patients' complaints during a phone call, in an e-mail, or in a video conversation are critical to assessment.

Benefits of telenursing include the ability to provide cost-effective care for patients at home or in rural areas and elimination of barriers associated with time zones. However, nurses must be cognizant of the differences between face-to-face or video dialogue and strictly electronic communication. Recall from Chapter 1 that 80% to 90% of communication is nonverbal. This can result in significant limitations with texting and e-mailing because it is difficult to impart feeling or tone. How a message is composed and how it is received may involve emotions and relationship factors that are not clear in the text and emoticons. For example, consider the following text from a nurse to an out-of-state patient: "Your test results are positive. Please call for more details." This seems to be a clear directive, but it doesn't take into consideration the potential emotion on the part of the patient and may be seen by the receiver as cold and impersonal.

A lack of face-to-face communication becomes even more critical when nurses are attempting to assess a patient. When a nurse sees a patient in person, she is constantly making visual assessments. Facial color and grimacing aren't visible through text or e-mail (or even over the telephone), and there is no opportunity for skin contact to allow for a rough temperature read.

Communicating Digitally in the Traditional Workplace

In traditional healthcare settings, digital communication also plays a major role. Tablets and smartphones are now everyday tools used by nurses and their colleagues. Nurses text colleagues when they are running late and send e-mails with shift schedules. Facebook and LinkedIn are used to make professional connections. Perhaps some nursing students and instructors are using smartphones and tablets to gain immediate access to current pharmacology information, treatment guidelines, or patient teaching materials that are specific to questions that come up in classrooms or clinical rotations. Google Plus offers opportunities to join or form groups of nursing colleagues and provides technology to hold virtual meetings with up to 10 visible participants online. Online forums exist on which common interests are discussed and often moderated. Blogging provides any nurse who has a message and wants to write the ability to post her words online. Twitter also allows information to be shared by nurses with people all over the world. For example, Brittney Wilson (2014), an informatics nurse known for educating nurses about health information technology, has used Twitter and written blog entries to help her cope with bullying she experienced as a nurse. She has commented that communicating with other nurses has helped her to feel supported.

Privacy and Ethical Issues

Whatever form of digital communication they are using at any given time and for whatever reason, nurses have an ethical and legal responsibility to maintain patient privacy at all times, and failure to do so could result in serious disciplinary action for breach of confidentiality and unprofessional or unethical conduct. Digital communication has created some blurry boundaries around privacy, so it is imperative that nurses be vigilant about appropriate use. In general, any information that nurses have about patients results from the fact that they have professional relationships with them. This information does not belong to nurses, nor is it theirs to share, except with other healthcare professionals who are also caring for the patient or with people who the patient has authorized to be given this information. In addition, talking about patients, whether identified by name or not, with others outside the healthcare team is inappropriate. The same goes for making unprofessional or disparaging remarks about colleagues, organizations, and so on. Any information, pictures, or videos that are shared on social media can never be considered private. After information is shared digitally, on some level, it can always be accessed. Students should recall and apply the goal of the therapeutic relationship discussed in Chapter 6 when using electronic media to share information with colleagues about patients as well as maintaining a professional demeanor with all forms of interprofessional communication. Recommendations from the National Council of State Boards of Nursing (2011) for nurses about the appropriate use of social media are consistent with the general guidelines given here.

It is also worth mentioning that maintaining a respectful presence online is an example of professional demeanor and important even when nurses are not at work. There are examples of unprofessional behavior among nurses online, such as using profanity or describing medical procedures using crude language. Such expressions, whether intended or not, bring unfavorable light on the profession.

Confident Voices

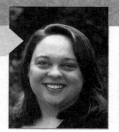

Erica MacDonald, RN, BSN, MSN
Nurse Educator

Healthcare Transparency and Online Diligence for Nurses
Major changes are occurring in our healthcare system and our society. The evolutionary change of the healthcare land-scape is being driven by social polices and technologic advances. While new technology provides the tools for medical teams to save lives, it also has resulted in healthcare transparency. For example, the public now has online access to resources such as electronic health records (EHRs) and healthcare reviews.

Potential healthcare customers "shop" for healthcare services by conducting Internet searches to review healthcare quality grades, facility amenities, and professional reputations. It would be wise for healthcare professionals to regularly monitor their online presence. They also should learn how to effectively communicate by electronic means in order to protect their professional reputation and comply with HIPPA. Something as seemingly insignificant as a text message has the potential to "go viral" with the click of a button and could produce positive or negative results.

Indeed, reputations can be ruined or greatly enhanced by the manner in which a person communicates using technology in the professional setting as well as in his or her personal life. Electronic communication used in the healthcare setting commonly includes e-mail, text messages, video conference, documentation within the EHR, and fax. It is not always a part of most healthcare professionals' job duties to use social media; however, personal use can still affect a professional's image.

Effective electronic communication begins with the knowledge that after a person posts a message or clicks send, it is potentially accessible for eternity. It cannot be taken back. After writing a message that is intended for any type of electronic communication including social media, use the following three-step review process before sending:

1. **Read the post or message slowly and edit it if needed.** Does it contain spelling or grammatical errors? Is the message clear and concise? Does it adequately convey the intended message?
2. **Imagine that the message was received instead of sent.** Does the tone of the message come across as friendly, approachable, and professional? Is there any way that the receiver could misconstrue or take offense to the message? Could this message be taken out of context or cause potential harm?
3. **After careful evaluation, send the message.**

Continued

Confident Voices—cont'd

In addition to using this three-step process, effective social media and electronic communication includes online reputation management, which can be done in the following ways:

- Using Google Alerts to monitor keywords, names, and companies online
- Developing a plan to deal with negative mentions or reviews online
- Cleaning up all social media profiles by taking down all nonprofessional content so that it is not easily accessible
- Enhancing your professional reputation by sharing reliable, factual, and educational healthcare content
- Learning how to competently use social media and knowing the differences in each platform's privacy settings

Healthcare workers also always need to protect patients, as afforded them by HIPAA. Nurses must do the following:

- **Never post pictures or information about a patient online or through any other form of electronic communication.** In fact, don't take pictures of your patients at all, even if you think that they will be unidentifiable.
- **Never discuss patient scenarios when using electronic communication, even if a patient's name is removed.** The nature of some injuries or surgeries could still potentially identify a patient.
- **Follow work or student polices regarding electronic communication.** Know the procedure to be followed if a data breach occurs, such as a mobile device being lost or stolen.

If questions arise regarding how a patient's Protected Health Information (PHI) is being safeguarded in the work or school setting, seek answers. Although healthcare is moving toward total transparency and healthcare professionals are increasingly under the public's microscope, diligence must be used to protect a patient's privacy. Following these simple guidelines will help protect healthcare professionals and their patients.

Biography

Erica MacDonald, RN, BSN, MSN, is a nurse educator as well as a nurse entrepreneur. Her nursing clinical experience includes the specialties of neonatal intensive care, postpartum, well baby, and labor and delivery. Her academic passion is the specialty of nurse entrepreneurship, which supports and encourages nurses to practice to the fullest extent of their education, licensing, and training. To find out more about Erica's mission, teaching, or business, visit her website at www.selfemployednurse.com.

CASE STUDY

Jeremy and Sandy are nursing students in their second year of a baccalaureate nursing program. They both have an interest in emergency nursing and decide to start a blog. They call the blog "Emergency Room Futures for Student Nurses" and take turns writing posts about new information in emergency nursing as well as their own aspirations and experiences. Many of their fellow students and a few faculty members follow their blog, and there is a growing audience of students in other programs in the United States and even internationally. One post they cowrite is critical of the BCMA system being used in the emergency department of one of their clinical sites. They are careful not to mention the facility by name but refer to examples of workarounds being used there. In one instance, they mention a nurse who carried several patients' bar codes on her belt and caused some confusion in the treatment of three family members who were brought in following a motor vehicle crash. One of the blog's readers is married to one of the nurses who works in the facility, and he shows it to his wife. A faculty member e-mails Jeremy and Sandy, telling them to delete the blog post. Sandy obliges immediately.

Discussion Questions

1. In what way could Jeremy and Sandy have used their blog in a better manner to provide constructive feedback about the BCMA system and the workarounds they observed?
2. How do you think a family member or friend of the victims of the motor vehicle crash might have felt if they read the article? What about other members of the community where the hospital is located? Can you think of any other possible ramifications?
3. What course of action do you think the dean of nursing should take in response to this incident? Support your opinion.

SUMMARY

Individuals and leaders must collaborate and engage in open, honest, and respectful communication to optimize the application of health information technology in the interests of patient safety and workforce satisfaction. With rapid advances in health information technology and digital communication, using the basic principles of assertiveness and listening will help to drive technology to meet the goal of patient-safe, cost-effective, and timely care. Effective communication will help avoid misunderstandings that may arise when using new software systems and is critical in maintaining patient privacy at all times.

Reflection Questions

1. Given what you've read in this chapter about EMR, what suggestions do you have that would maximize its benefits and minimize its problems?

2. How would you handle a situation at work or in a clinical rotation in which members of the nursing staff are skipping steps in the BCMA process? Have you ever observed workarounds by nursing staff around any other technology? If so, did you talk with any of the nurses to find out why they developed the workaround?

3. Have you ever been hurt or angry because of an e-mail message? Do you think you made any assumptions or interpreted the message in a way it may not have been intended? Did you or could you have taken steps to clarify and share your experience?

4. What social media programs do you use? Have you ever shared something that was intended for a particular group or person and have it end up in others' mailboxes or on their social media pages?

References

Boonstra, A., & Broekhuis, M. (2010). Barriers to the acceptance of electronic medical records by physicians from systematic review to taxonomy and interventions. *BMC Health Services Research, 10*(231). Retrieved from www.biomedcentral.com/1472-6963/10/231

Buchanan, N. S. (1984). *Evolution of a hospital information system.* Springfield, VA: National Technical Information Service.

Centers for Medicare and Medicaid Services. (2014). 2014 Definition stage 1 of meaningful use. Retrieved from www.cms.gov/Regulations-and-Guidance/Legislation/EHRIncentivePrograms/Meaningful_Use.html

Gooder, V. (2011). Nurses' perceptions of a (BCMA) bar-coded medication administration system: A case-control study. *OJNI: Online Journal of Nursing Informatics, 15*(2). Retrieved from ojni.org/issues/?p=703

Institute of Medicine. (2012). *Health IT and patient safety: Building safer systems for better care.* Washington, DC: The National Academies Press.

Koppel, R., Wetterneck, T., Telles, J. L., & Karsh, B-T. (2008). Workarounds to barcode medication administration systems: Their occurrences, causes, and threats to patient safety. *Journal of the American Medical Informatics Association, 15*(4), 408–423.

National Council of State Boards of Nursing. (2011). Brochure A nurse's guide to the use of social media. Retrieved from https://www.ncsbn.org/NCSBN_SocialMedia.pdf

Pennsylvania Patient Safety Authority. (2008). Medication errors occurring with the use of bar-code administration technology. *Pennsylvania Patient Safety Advisory 5*(4), 122–126. Retrieved from patientsafetyauthority.org/ADVISORIES/AdvisoryLibrary/2008/Dec5%284%29/Pages/122.aspx

Thede, L. (2012). Informatics: Where is it? *OJIN: The Online Journal of Issues in Nursing, 17*(1), 10. Retrieved from www.nursingworld.org/MainMenuCategories/ANAMarketplace/ANAPeriodicals/OJIN/Columns/Informatics/Informatics-Where-Is-It.html

Wilson, B. (2014). *The nerdy nurse's guide to technology.* Indianapolis, IN: Sigma Theta Tau International.

CHAPTER 15

Preparing for Leadership

- Discuss the reasoning for increased focus on leadership competencies among nurse professionals
- Identify communication and emotional intelligence skills necessary for developing related competencies promoted by the American Nurses Association Leadership Institute
- Describe three leadership models that are prevalent in current nursing practice and literature
- Identify six leadership styles that nurse leaders can use in appropriate circumstances
- Demonstrate application of communication and leadership skills in situations requiring delegation and conflict management

KEY TERMS

- Servant leadership
- Transformational leadership
- Complexity leadership
- Delegation
- Conflict management

All practicing nurses must be prepared to take on leadership roles and responsibilities, and leadership skills are requisite in patient advocacy and in setting limits and priorities for healthy work–life balance and lifelong learning. In this chapter, students will explore common leadership styles and prevalent leadership trends and models in nursing. In addition, they will examine leadership competencies with a focus on developing the communication skills and emotional intelligence necessary for delegation and conflict management. To begin, students will learn why there is a new and growing focus in the profession on developing the leadership abilities of nurses.

PREPARING NURSE LEADERS

Nursing leadership roles have long been a part of organizational, educational, and professional development. As a student, sharing knowledge and resources with others, accepting constructive feedback, asking questions during clinical rotation meetings, and forming study groups all provide leaderships opportunities. When licensed and practicing, nurses may automatically be positioned in leadership roles, such as a charge nurse supervising nursing assistants in a long-term care facility. As careers unfold and depending on interests, skills, and organizational needs, many nurses will have additional opportunities to develop their leadership skills (e.g., leading a discussion in a team meeting). Some nurses may go on to obtain advanced degrees in order to become leaders in a particular clinical specialty, education, policy-making, or self-employed businesses.

Although the opportunities for leadership have always been there, preparing nurses for leadership has in recent years taken on even greater importance. The current focus on nurse leadership has arisen out of concerns for the welfare of the healthcare workforce and the need for nurse leaders to advocate for and build healthy workplaces. In their review of nursing literature and discussion of leadership skills, educators Rose Sherman and Elizabeth Pross (2010) make a compelling case for promoting nurse leadership in efforts to improve staff satisfaction, retention, patient outcomes, and organizational performance.

The impetus for preparing nurses for leadership has also been fortified by the Institute of Medicine's (IOM, 2011) report, *The Future of Nursing: Leading Change, Advancing Health*. The report highlights the value that nurses bring to healthcare in terms of prevention, management of chronic illness, and direct interfaces with patients along all continuums of care. The report was found to be complementary to the Institute for Healthcare Improvement's Triple Aim Initiative (2014) for improving patient experience, improving the health of populations, and reducing the per capita cost of healthcare.

To best capitalize on the expertise of nurses, the IOM report recommends that the healthcare system "[p]repare and enable nurses to lead change to advance health. Nurses, nursing education programs, and nursing associations should prepare the nursing workforce to assume leadership positions across all levels, while public, private, and governmental health care decision-makers should ensure that leadership positions are available to and filled by nurses" (IOM, 2011, p. S-12).

LEADERSHIP COMPETENCIES

In response to the call for better preparation of nurse leaders, the number of programs and resources for nurse leadership has been steadily growing. Susan Hassmiller, a senior advisor for nursing for the Robert Wood Johnson Foundation and study director for the project resulting in the *Future of Nursing* report, and Julia Truelove, a nursing student at the University of Virginia School of Nursing, created a comprehensive list of nurse leadership programs available to nursing students and professional nurses within the categories of public health, education, clinical specialty, business, and research (Hassmiller & Truelove, 2014).

As well, the American Nurses Association (ANA) Leadership Institute (2013) offers and continues to develop a variety of programs designed to build leadership competencies. Within the ANA programs, three progressive leadership tracks are addressed—emerging, developing, and advanced—and within each of those are three domains—leading self, leading others, and leading the organization. There are competencies and behaviors associated with each domain for each level of leadership.

Self-image, self-awareness, and self-management are competencies listed under the domain of leading self. These competencies fall under emotional intelligence (discussed in Chapter 2) and require the ability to reflect and act out of respect for one's needs, limits, and desires. These elements are necessary for presenting a professional demeanor and role-modeling conduct that reflects respect and confidence. Knowing one's own capabilities is directly related to being able to delegate and supervise, which is necessary for safe and cost-effective frontline care.

Competencies related to the domain of leading others include emotional intelligence, respectful listening (Chapter 3), assertiveness (Chapter 4), team development (Chapter 10), diversity (Chapter 13), and conflict management (discussed later in this chapter). Bedside nurses are constantly weaving in and out of individual- and team-oriented tasks that require navigating conflict, getting help, and supervising nurse assistants, all of which require the knowledge, skills, and attitudes related to leading others.

Leading the organization competencies include those related to systems thinking (Chapter 11), change management (Chapter 12), and promotion of the organizational vision and strategy. The first two competencies have their roots in the assertiveness and the respectful listening required for setting limits and respecting others, and they are essential for the dynamic learning, conflict management, quality improvement, and teamwork that make up human systems. Promotion of a vision and strategic planning requires effective communication and must take into consideration organizational culture, including implicit and explicit norms that guide workplace behaviors (Chapter 10), patient care outcomes, and organizational goals. Strategic planning is commonly done at more advanced leadership levels, yet all levels of leaders can appreciate its value.

LEADERSHIP MODELS IN NURSING

To be effective, leaders must have certain characteristics, including expertise in a field, an ability to influence others, an authority over others, and a collaborative relationship with others. Although there may be common characteristics in leadership, there is a wide range of leadership models. The particular model someone uses depends on individual preferences and strengths, educational opportunities and requirements, and an organization's culture and mission. Several models of leadership are prominent in current nursing literature.

Servant Leadership

Servant leadership emphasizes collaboration, community, and inclusion in decision making, and it also promotes respect of self and others. Servant leaders achieve results for their organizations by attending to the needs of those they serve (Greenleaf & Spears, 1977). A nurse who is a servant leader seeks to support the needs of her staff and continually asks how she can help them solve their problems and promote their personal development. Effective communication skills are critical in this philosophy because nurse leaders will need to ask staff what they need in order to get out on time, manage a patient assignment, or meet personal goals. Self- and situational awareness are required because it is extremely helpful to know one's own limits and be aware of what is going on with others, including patients, staff, and physicians. Nurse leaders practicing within this model also need to remember to take care of themselves so that they are able to sustain long-term and healthy leadership roles.

Transformational Leadership

Transformational leadership was originally introduced by historian and political scientist James Macgregor Burns (1978) as a process whereby "one or more persons engage with others in such a way that leaders and followers help each other to advance to a higher level of morale and motivation" (p. 20). Transformational leaders are able to guide major change and inspire commitment, both of which are necessary in today's rapidly changing healthcare environment. Quite different from the top-down hierarchical approach of command-and-control in which leaders dictate to followers what to do, when, and how, a transformational philosophy promotes growth and is dependent on the quality of relationships. Transformational leadership is a primary component of the American Nurses Credentialing Center's (2014) recommendations for hospitals wishing to achieve Magnet designation, a program that recognizes healthcare facilities that demonstrate excellence and "requires vision, influence, clinical knowledge, and a strong expertise relating to professional nursing practice" (para. 6). Communication skills necessary in transformational leadership include articulating a compelling vision, listening to and understanding staff, clinical motivational interviewing, advocating for resources, and setting limits.

Complexity Leadership

Complexity leadership is a style in which the leader "is in the midst of the action; cultivating relationships; accepting feedback, tolerating messy, uncertain situations; and seeking diverse opinions, all the while staying centered and self-reflective" (Crowell, 2011, p. 3). To lead with this approach, nurses must understand that hospital units or healthcare facilities are complex adaptive systems, and they must have the communication skills and emotional intelligence to create an environment in which both individuals and teams are collaborating for optimal patient outcomes. Leaders practicing this philosophy will create a positive culture and inspire a vision so that desired outcomes will emerge, and to do so there must be mutual trust between leaders and followers. There also needs to be support that complements or strengthens the properties of complex adaptive systems, including adaptability, the butterfly effect, and diversity. Such support might include training in giving and receiving feedback, role-modeling a high regard for diversity, and encouraging and listening to new ideas, all of which can contribute to quality improvement.

Collaborative leadership is another model that is very similar to complexity leadership, in that it focuses on teamwork and interpersonal relationships. It also is built on authentic leadership, which emphasizes personal growth and an honest reflection on one's own life story.

Confident Voices

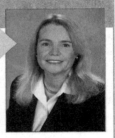

Rose O. Sherman, EdD, RN, NEA-BC, FAAN
Professor and Director

How to Build a Sense of Community in Your Workplace

Feeling a sense of community in the workplace and establishing close relationships with coworkers have been closely linked to job satisfaction and staff retention. This is not surprising when you consider that staff members may spend as much time with one another at work as they do with family members. For some staff, work may be the only community in which they participate, so having a sense of community at work matters even more. Building a sense of community is the responsibility of all nurses, not just those in leadership roles. Yet this can prove challenging in some environments. Following are seven ways that you can foster a sense of community on your unit.

1. **Remind everyone about the importance of purpose in your work and values.**
   A key element in forming a strong sense of community is a shared vision among members in the purpose of work and common values. We sometimes

make assumptions that there is a shared sense of purpose and values among staff, but this may not be case. To build a sense of community, you need to collectively discuss issues such as the mission of your organization and what should guide everyday behavior.

2. **Be inclusive.** To build strong communities, everyone must feel like a valued member. This includes all who contribute to the goals of the unit, including interdisciplinary team members, housekeeping, and engineering. Take the time to learn the names of your coworkers. Avoid forming cliques and openly arranging social events that clearly exclude some staff members.

3. **Value individual differences.** Part of the joy of being human is the recognition that we are all different and have unique gifts. To build community, we need to recognize these individual differences and capitalize on each person's strengths.

4. **Encourage an environment of trust.** Strong communities at work are built in an environment of trust. You can help foster this trust by refusing to engage in gossip, speculation, or criticism of others when they are not present.

5. **Urge your coworkers to tell their stories.** It might surprise you how little nursing staff members know about one another in some environments. Help staff on your unit to learn more about one another and what is important to them in their work. Huddles and staff meetings can be great opportunities for sharing. Take the time to learn about the lives of your coworkers, such as when their birthdays are and the names of their children. In today's environment, many staff live alone and may not have close family or friends.

6. **Embrace conflict.** Conflict is an inevitable part of teamwork. In nursing environments where unit staff may see each other infrequently, conflict can build and go unresolved. Recognize that conflict is part of being a member of a community, but also actively look for ways to reduce tension. There may be times when there is a need to agree to disagree.

7. **Look for opportunities to celebrate.** Celebrating holidays and special events such as New Year's Day, birthdays, and staff achievements all help to build a sense of community among staff. The importance of sharing meals cannot be underestimated as a way of fostering a sense of belonging. Participation in community events such as charity walks or drives can be a great way to develop staff camaraderie.

In helping to make your workplace more enjoyable, you will boost employee morale and improve staff satisfaction. A sense of community energizes staff, reduces absenteeism, and ultimately improves patient care.

Continued

Confident Voices—cont'd

Recommended Reading

Manion, J., & Bartholomew, K. (2004). Community in the workplace: A proven retention strategy. *Journal of Nursing Administration, 34*(1), 46–53.

Sherman, R. O. (2013). Building a sense of community on nursing units. *American Nurse Today, 8*(3), 32–34.

Biography

Dr. Rose Sherman, EdD, RN, NEA-BC, FAAN, is the director of the Nursing Leadership Institute and a professor at the Christine E. Lynn College of Nursing at Florida Atlantic University (FAU). Before joining the faculty at FAU, Dr. Sherman had a 25-year nursing leadership career with the Department of Veterans Affairs. She has published extensively in nursing journals and speaks nationally and internationally on nursing leadership topics. She is also the editor of a popular blog, Emerging RN Leader (www.emergingrnleader.com), designed to help emerging nurse leaders on their leadership journey.

LEADERSHIP STYLES

Although models provide framework and theory about the role and responsibility of leadership, styles describe different approaches or ways of behaving that leaders can use in order to accomplish their mission. Different leadership styles are appropriate for different circumstances. Terminology for and descriptions of leadership styles vary among theorists, so for the purposes of this chapter, the leadership styles described all come from the book, *Primal Leadership: Realizing the Power of Emotional Intelligence* (Goleman, Boyatzis, & McKee, 2013).

The goal, at this stage, should not be to master each style, but rather to be aware of when they may or may not be helpful. This knowledge will also be useful in exploring and developing related foundational skills necessary for delegation and conflict management (discussed shortly).

Visionary

The visionary style of leadership emphasizes the ideal future in terms of desirable goals, outcomes, and general direction that an organization is going in. It is most appropriate when a group, team, or organization needs a new focus: "Visionary leaders articulate where a group is going, but not how it will get there—setting people free to innovate, experiment, take calculated risks" (Goleman, Boyatzis, & McKee, 2013, p. 57). For example, the nurse in charge of one or more nursing assistants might articulate a vision related to the next 8 hours with staff: "I know we've got some challenges ahead, but I'd like to see us pull off a great shift together. Are you ready?"

Coaching

The coaching style focuses on developing individuals by showing them how to improve their performance and helping to connect their goals to those of the team. Coaching is most effective "with employees who show initiative and want more professional development" (Goleman,

Boyatzis, & McKee, 2013, p. 61). This is generally a useful approach when nurses have established a respected relationship with staff because it requires a willingness to participate from the leader *and* staff member. Supportive and encouraging feedback is necessary as well as more difficult constructive feedback: "I notice you are doing a great job helping Mrs. Stevens with her shower. She seems much calmer now with your reassuring and gentle approach. I also noticed that you went to the linen cart several times and wonder if you might have saved yourself some time with a little more planning. What are your thoughts?"

Affiliative

The affiliative style emphasizes the importance of teamwork and creating positive interpersonal relationships. Attributes of this style include role-modeling and respectful listening as well as asserting an unwillingness to participate in gossip—all elements that will contribute to healthy dynamics on a nursing unit even if they cause some initial tension. "When leaders are being affiliative they focus on the emotional needs of employees, even over work goals" (Goleman, Boyatzis, & McKee, 2013, p. 65). It should be noted that on a unit with a toxic culture, an affiliative approach would not be advised without more substantial leadership training or very close supervision. Such volatile dynamics inherently complicate application of this style, making it challenging even for the most seasoned nurse leader. Ideally, getting support to address concerns about a toxic culture before trying to enforce changes makes the most sense. Until that can happen, nurse leaders should proceed with caution if attempting to use this leadership style under these circumstances because forcing teamwork on nurses who have old resentments between each other may compromise care: "Mary and Bill, you two haven't worked together much, so let's put you on a team on South Wing. Bill, you've been doing a great job with the new stocking process, and Mary, you've made some great progress with Mrs. Granopolis. See what you can learn from each other. And remember, no gossiping!"

Democratic

A democratic style engages everyone's knowledge and skills and creates a group commitment to the intended goals. It works best when there is uncertainty about goals, there is a sense that individuals need to be heard in order to engage them in a particular project, or "the leader needs ideas from able employees" (Goleman, Boyatzis, & McKee, 2013, p. 67). This style requires inviting input, considering it, and being decisive about how to go forward all in a short amount of time. For example, a charge nurse can gather staff for a quick conversation and invite input: "We've got one person out sick so that is going to require us all to work a little harder. Let's take a couple minutes. What concerns or ideas do you have?" Once asked, nurse leaders must make sure that everyone has a chance to provide input: "Sally, we haven't heard from you. What are your thoughts?" Someone might suggest coordinating meal breaks with supplying the linens or ask for help at a certain time, both of which allow for more thoughtful planning that may make a difference and at the very least will help form the team.

Pacesetting

With a pacesetting style, the leader sets the pace of activity. The leader using this style is typically "obsessive about doing things better and faster, and asks the same of everyone" (Goleman, Boyatzis, & McKee, 2013, p. 72). Healthcare facilities are often bustling with urgent activity, but leaders should be cautious about setting expectations that everyone work at maximum speed every minute. This will likely lead to resentment, burnout, and unsafe practices. More than the other styles, this approach comes with the expectation that everyone should role-model the leader, which can be can be hard to enforce on a group of very different and independent people. Nevertheless, this style is useful when the need arises to speed up, such as when a quick response is needed to a cardiac code: "Code Blue, room 12B! Kara, get the code cart. Tracey, page the rapid response team. Mike, you and I will start CPR." This style can even work in the opposite situation, when the pace needs to slow down for a short period, such as taking time to accept the death of a long-term resident: "Let's stop for a minute and remember Mrs. Haberif and her family."

Commanding

The classic model of military-style leadership is the commanding style. A commanding leader is one who "erodes people's spirits and the pride and satisfaction they take in their work—the very things that motivate most high-performing workers" (Goleman, Boyatzis, & McKee, 2013, p. 77). Despite its negative consequences, the commanding style is very common in healthcare organizations overall because quick, clear, decision making is frequently warranted. It is also useful in circumstances when there is no time for discussion or when discussion is unlikely to be productive. When supervising nurse assistants, nurse leaders may be bombarded with requests to have particular patient assignments, work with a friend, or take a break at a certain time. These conversations can be very time-consuming, and efforts to make one person happy will most likely make another angry. The best approach is to validate concerns, be as fair as possible, be decisive, and always keep patient care as the priority: "I hear your frustrations about working with Mr. Lantini. I understand that he requires a lot of patience"—a pause here is a very important moment of validation that should be separate from the next statement—"but I am not going to change the assignment for several reasons, one of which is that he seems to feel safe with you. We can talk more about your concerns at the end of the shift." A more democratic or affiliative discussion might be helpful later to ensure that additional staff are introduced to and trained to work with this patient or other difficult patients.

Daniel Goleman and his colleagues (2013) warn about the use of commanding and pacesetting leadership styles: "In America today, many medical organizations are facing a crisis of leadership in part because the culture of medicine has favored pacesetting and commanding styles. These styles are appropriate in say the operating or emergency rooms. But their predominance means that many medical people that rise to positions of leadership have had too few chances to learn a fuller repertoire of styles" (p. 77). Although this author would qualify this statement to advise that these styles are appropriate at times in these areas, the overall point is well taken and consistent with discussion about toxic hierarchy in Chapter 10.

FUNDAMENTALS OF DELEGATION

Although delegation of tasks can occur among peers, most frequently this responsibility falls to nurses in leadership positions. **Delegation** requires communicating effectively in order to give instruction to others. It also requires that nurse leaders practice situational awareness and follow-up to ensure delegated tasks are performed safely, timely, and compassionately.

Giving instruction to others requires clear and firm language and resisting the urge to ask when, in fact, there is little choice involved. For example, consider the difference between the following requests:

"Would you mind seeing what Mrs. Santiago wants?"

Or

"Answer that light, please."

Consultant Commentary

Janine was a first-year staff RN at a rehabilitation hospital when she contacted me for some short-term leadership coaching at her unit manager's suggestion. Six months into her full-time evening position, she was very exhausted and frustrated and was considering leaving not only her job, but also the profession itself. She worked on a subacute rehabilitation wing that included eight rooms with two beds each, so she typically provided nursing care for 16 patients who were on the unit anywhere from 1 to 4 weeks. Janine had two nursing assistants to supervise, and there were five who rotated through her unit; three had been employees of the hospital for more than 5 years, and the other two only came to the facility in the last year. Through our first phone conversation and, with Janine's permission, a talk with her manager, I gained a fairly good understanding of some of the difficult interpersonal dynamics she was experiencing in relation to the assistants and aides she was supervising. She acknowledged that she wanted the staff to like her and was finding it hard to say "no" when the assistants asked to take cigarette breaks. She noticed that staff members were bickering among themselves and seemed to be asking for more and more of these brief breaks. There was also one assistant who frequently complained to her about the others. One especially busy evening, a patient had fallen when, unknown to Janine, both the assistants had left the floor. The patient was fine, but Janine received a verbal warning about the incident. She was unsure how things got to be so out of control and what she should do about it.

First, I told Janine that she was going to need to set some new boundaries with the staff and that turning this around would take some time. She was willing to do the work, and her unit manager offered to help in any way she could. I reassured her that, although it would be a difficult process, I felt she could do it, and with some guidance over the next few weeks, she did change her leadership style. First, she and her manager scheduled a meeting with all of the assistants. In this meeting, Janine announced that she was making a change in her supervisory style and had some new expectations for staff. She spoke clearly with a confident voice as we had practiced: "Ms. Phillips's fall last month was a wake-up call for me. I was all alone on the floor and hadn't realized one of you was on meal break when I had given the other an okay to take a quick break. I blame myself for not being more in charge. Historically, I've been too flexible about breaks and assignments, and I'm not going to do that anymore. I expect you all to work together respectfully and efficiently. You don't have to like each other, or me, but we have to work together to provide safe and compassionate care. Do you have any questions?" With this conversation, she set new limits, and over the next few weeks, she worked very diligently to maintain them. This involved saying "no" to breaks or changing assignments to make staff happy. It also required her to step in and give feedback to one of the long-term assistants who had a habit of telling her negative things about the other assistants, such as their being "too slow" or "too lazy": "Charlie, I appreciate different strengths about each of you. If you are concerned about the way one of your colleagues is behaving and don't feel comfortable talking with them privately, we can schedule a meeting with the manager. It is important that we are able to provide safe, quality care individually and together." Gradually, the assistants came to respect her leadership, and Janine developed some very important skills. Eventually, she was able to be more affiliative with her staff and feel more positive about her work.

The second instruction is polite and clear but also commanding. Some nurses may feel this is being bossy or will lead to others disliking them, but clear instruction actually helps others to be successful in their jobs and will help to earn trust and respect from all team members. However, effective delegation must leave room for dialogue and conflict when a colleague or support staff feels unable or is unwilling to take on a delegated task. It is also important to note that a supervisor delegating a task or procedure to someone who is unlicensed or a volunteer retains responsibility for the task being done correctly and safely, whereas a task accepted by a licensed peer or manager will become that person's responsibility.

Delegation is an important aspect of providing cost-effective and safe care. Besides that it financially costs the healthcare organization more for the nurse to do a simple task such as getting linens than for a nurse assistant to do the same task, and assistants should be properly used to complete certain tasks in order to keep nurses available for the tasks they have been trained to do. As well, nurse leaders who do not delegate properly to other nurses, aides, and assistants run the risk for burning out, resulting in potentially unsafe practices.

Confident Voices

Nance Goldstein, PhD, ACC
Industrial Economist and Resident Scholar

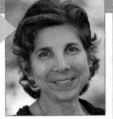

Engaging Millennial Nurses in a VUCA World: How Every Nurse Leader Can Help

Seismic changes now rock hospitals and healthcare decision making. Nurses and nurse leaders face this daily: Everyone must get involved now to deliver better patient value at lower cost. But no one really knows what that means in a VUCA (*volatile, uncertain, complex,* and *ambiguous*) world. One thing, though, is essential: Today's nurses must coordinate patient care across boundaries of all kinds—organizations, providers, and other differences. Crucially, the changes call on nurses to lead and support 20-something clinicians. With more than half of all nurses planning to retire soon, Millennials must become the seasoned experts patients need. Yet they feel frustrated and disrespected—and they want to leave. That leads to predictions of unprecedented clinical shortages if healthcare organizations do not engage younger clinicians. Nurse leaders urgently need to communicate with 20-somethings to retain them to improve the future of healthcare.

Nurse leaders and nurse colleagues who communicate the following intentions and information will reduce workplace conflict and anxiety and likely retain clinicians of all kinds:

1. **Tell your staff you expect them to respect others . . . and make sure you offer them yours.** Ask for your staff to treat others with respect and to come to work planning to contribute. Then model this for them. Show them you understand and welcome differences in values, experience, and perspectives.

Communicate practices, priorities, performance needs, and decision-making criteria clearly. This helps staff to see their roles and performance targets and to feel that managers treat them with fairness.

2. **Listen so that your staff truly hears you.** Listening—truly listening—is the secret ingredient to others hearing you. Listening to what 20-somethings care about and what they're asking enables you to communicate in ways that will connect you. When 20-somethings ask you a question, they expect a real answer. That's how they were raised. "Because I said so" answers alienate them and slow down their learning. Although the situation may not allow much time to answer, effective managers assure their readiness to answer later. Too often, younger clinicians get snubbed for asking and never get answers to their questions.

3. **Discover something you admire in each staff person.** This nips one's preconceptions right in the bud. Forge a relationship with each staff person so that you know what each knows, needs, and offers. This helps you see the person in front of you, not his youth or your assumptions about his age. Knowing one another gives even brief conversations context and continuity. It builds the trust that is key in fast, high-risk decision-making environments. Create a lot of face-to-face opportunities to get to know your staff and to build relationships. Recent research discussion forums, hot topics discussions, and more formal periodic one-to-one nonpunitive meetings all help leaders and staff learn about one another.

4. **Motivate them (yes, that's your job).** Communicate the organization's vision to your staff members and their role in it. Repeat this often so that everyone sees the path you are on together and the behaviors that are key to hospital success. Magnetic managers make and communicate their decisions in ways that incorporate young people's interests and concerns as well as the hospital's. This proves particularly important because 20-somethings tend to look "up" for motivation. Regularly ask staff of all ages about their ideas and concerns, and then create ways, both informal and formal, for each clinician to contribute. These vital behaviors show the way things will be done. Also communicate to your boss your eagerness to find opportunities for your staff to learn and development their futures. Ask for training, rotation, shadowing, and conference opportunities. And bring them to your meetings where people plan for the big picture issues and needs.

5. **Meet with each staff person to plan his or her future.** Sit down periodically to identify professional goals and useful learning opportunities, performance milestones, and resulting compensation. This both clarifies performance expectations

Continued

and tells the staff how they can advance within the hospital system. If you do not communicate your expectations clearly, younger clinicians won't know how they can create their careers. They'll feel stuck, and they'll leave for another opportunity.

6. **Cultivate their professional futures with every conversation.** Finding opportunities for 20-somethings to grow is your job. Right now, they don't believe you care. They say that hospitals do this poorly. Frame every hallway conversation, e-mail, and decision as part of their professional development. Offer frequent, informal comment on their performance consistently so that they know what they are doing right and not just what they are doing wrong. "Feed-forward" reinforces what a person is doing right and offers ways to improve. It's honest, specific, right away, fair, and constructive. Its importance cannot be overstated. It improves staff performance, motivates, and reduces conflict. They expect it, and they're lost without it.

Showing 20-somethings there's a future they want in healthcare is not a choice. Young people offer vital, valuable qualities. Their desire to learn, experience in collaboration, and abilities to improve communication and care processes using information technologies are central to improving hospital performance.

Nurses, nurse case managers, and leaders have the perfect position to span these boundaries. Nurses are coordinators, boundary-spanning communicators, mediators, sense-makers, and visionaries from the point of view of the patient. This certainly asks you to step outside your comfort zone. However, individual leaders can dramatically improve the climate, often with simple intentions and communications. Our hospitals and patients depend on your succeeding.

Biography

Nance Goldstein, PhD, ACC, is as an industrial economist who has researched how information technologies changed jobs, skills, and working conditions in many industries, most recently in healthcare. She received research grants and commissions from the National Science Foundation and others and a Fellowship at Harvard's Radcliffe Institute for Advanced Study. She now helps frontline and middle hospital managers find new ways to respond to the continual torrent of difficult situations. She and her company, Working Wisely Group (workingwiselygroup.com), help clients become masterful motivators and leaders. As a resident scholar at Brandeis University WSRC (www.brandeis.edu/wsrc/scholars/profiles/goldstein.html), she brings current concepts and practices to enable them to face the VUCA world as managers who succeed for their staff, organizations, and themselves.

CONFLICT MANAGEMENT

Conflict occurs frequently in nurse practice settings. Differences in personalities, leadership styles, clinical expertise, patient or family expectations, available resources, goals among professional staff, and organizational priorities are just a few potential areas in which disagreements will come up. The degree of tension in a conflict varies with the nature of the topic, the history of the relationships, situational stress, the strength of communication skills, and the vulnerability of the stakeholders involved. In addition, differences in power and education held by healthcare professionals and paraprofessionals "creates disparity which also leads to conflict" (Education Career Articles, 2013).

Throughout this book, students have learned the essential skills for mastering **conflict management:** giving and receiving constructive feedback, assertiveness, and listening. However, the ability to demonstrate ownership about wants and needs, consider and validate other perspectives, and be genuinely curious are all more difficult when conflict arises. As well, effective communication and collaboration—critical for safe, cost-effective, patient-centered care—is vastly more challenging when people are feeling stressed and vulnerable or don't have the skills to confidently and respectfully express or listen to a perspective that is different from their own.

Managing conflict is never fun, and, although it gets less difficult with practice, it is seldom easy. But when conflict is managed properly, positive outcomes from conflict (e.g., developing new solutions, building trust, coexisting peacefully, optimizing creativity) are more likely than negative outcomes from avoiding or mismanaging conflict (e.g., resentment, mistrust, power struggles, and working in silos). Nurse leaders have several resources at their hands for learning to manage conflict. The Thomas-Kilmann Conflict Mode Instrument is one of the most popular research tools and describes five styles of conflict management: competing, collaborating, compromising, accommodating, and avoiding. It is frequently used in leadership training to help participants identify their predominant style and then develop a different style if necessary (Kilmann & Thomas, 1977; also see Kilmann, 2011, and Thomas & Kilmann, 1974).

Competing

A person practicing a competing style of conflict wants to dominate the conflict. To succeed with this style, one needs to hold power, which may come from one's organizational position, superior knowledge, persuasive ability, or a conflict with someone who acquiesces. A competing style is effective in some situations in nursing. For example, a staff nurse is reluctant to contact a patient's doctor regarding a patient's extreme pain. The manager decides to be forceful and clear in her effort to solve the conflict: She gives the nurse a stern look, grabs the phone, and uses the overhead page system to contact the physician. She is using assertiveness that is based on her clinical expertise for the best outcome for the patient. Circumstances like this are quite stressful for everyone and sometimes contribute to unprofessional behavior such as swearing, humiliating others, or even throwing things. A supervisor should speak with staff in a calmer manner after a crisis to ask what could have been done better, offer apologies when indicated, and review interpersonal dynamics to see how the situation could have been handled better: "I'm sorry about grabbing the phone and the look I gave you, but that patient's pain should have been addressed immediately. I want to schedule time with you to go over your pain management skills and give you more of a chance to explain your rationale."

Collaborating

Leaders using a collaborative style to manage conflicts try to meet the needs of all people involved, including themselves. These people can be highly assertive, but unlike competitive conflict managers, they cooperate effectively and acknowledge that everyone's perspective is important. This style is useful when needing to bring together a variety of viewpoints to get the best solution, when there have been previous conflicts in the group, or when the situation is too important for a simple compromise. For example, a nurse manager holds a brief unit meeting to ask staff nurses on the unit for their input about what is working and what is not with the new bar-coded medication administration process. Because several of the nurses have complained about the system, she wants to get a better grasp of the situation before considering solutions and discussing with senior management. Such a collaborative process is likely to yield solutions that are more effective.

However, a collaborative leadership style can become problematic in situations in which decisions need to be made quickly or when engaging with someone who isn't willing to collaborate on the issue. In those situations, as mentioned previously, a competitive style might be used initially and then followed by the collaborative approach when the timing and circumstances allow for it. However, this is hard to do in healthcare milieus where the next crisis is already happening and time available for debriefing is chronically eroded. People don't always have the chance to learn how their behaviors affect others, making collaborative conflict management impossible sometimes. Even though making the time for both is a challenge, the effort should never be completely ignored.

Compromising

The compromising style involves finding a solution to problems so that everyone is at least partly satisfied. Everyone gets something, but everyone will have to give up something, including the leader. An example of the best time to use a compromising conflict management style among nurses is during scheduling holiday or weekend sick call coverage. Conversations that involve everyone sharing their preferences while listening to others will hopefully result in a fair distribution of coverage and sacrifice. For example, a nurse manager is trying to schedule an in-service immediately following the 7:00 p.m. to 7:00 a.m. shift. All of the nurses agree to the timing, except for one nurse, who insists she cannot stay later. The nurse manager realizes it's not productive to move the in-service based on one's nurse's conflict. Instead, she proposes the following: "I can stay a little later and do it during your shift this afternoon. Will that work?" The compromising style can be problematic because everyone stands to lose something (Education Career Articles, 2013) and can become tiresome if leaders don't contribute to the compromising or individuals don't assert their needs into the situations. Burnout, tension, and resentment may permeate future teamwork, resulting in unsafe care and poor morale.

Accommodating

An accommodating style indicates a willingness to meet the needs of others at the expense of the leader's own needs. The accommodator often knows when to give in to others but can be persuaded to surrender a position even when it is not warranted. This person is not typically assertive and is cooperative almost to a fault. Accommodation is appropriate when the issues matter more to the other party, when peace is more valuable than winning, or when the leader wants to be in a position to collect on this "favor." For example, a nurse manager hears two overwhelmed nurses debating about who will take on the new admission from the emergency department. She decides to be accommodating and says, "Never mind, I'll go get him." If this manager has to ask one of these staff members to work overtime later in the shift, then her accommodation of them in the earlier situation may sway them to say "yes." However, leaders must realize that people do not always return favors, and overall this approach is unlikely to result in the best outcomes if used frequently. Further, nurse leaders who give up their own needs over and over again may end up burned out, suffering from compassion fatigue, or holding invisible resentments toward the people they supervise. A patient-centered approach to care must keep the needs of caregivers in mind in order to sustain healthy and safe care. Too often, there is a tendency to teach nurses to be assertive for patients, but not for themselves, and chronic accommodation is an unhealthy manifestation of this.

Avoiding

Supervisors who use an avoiding style seek to put off or evade the conflict entirely. Many leaders who are uncomfortable with conflict will delegate decisions or avoid conversations on controversial topics as much as possible. They may worry about hurting other people's feelings or feel insecure about their own opinions or expertise. These are not good reasons to avoid conflict. For example, a manager who puts a nurse on a particular weekend schedule to avoid dealing with a conflict that the nurse has with someone on the alternating weekend may be giving a message to staff that one way to switch weekend assignments is to be in conflict with others. Avoiding can be appropriate when a crisis is occurring, when the controversy is trivial, or when someone else is in a better position to solve the problem; sometimes avoiding an aggressive peer or physician is the wisest tactic. However, finding a way to address the conflict later through human resources or another avenue is equally important. It is not healthy for any individual, relationship, team, or organization to avoid conflict all the time. In order to maintain a positive organizational culture, leaders must find the time and place for giving and receiving constructive feedback. For relationships that are strained, whether involving two people or an entire team, efforts must be made to focus more intently on managing conflict.

CASE STUDY

Eliza is the nurse manager of an acute care geriatric psychiatric unit. One of her nurses, Ralph, has a patient on his unit who is extremely aggressive at times, but the physician has been reluctant to increase antipsychotic medication. For the past two weekends, Ralph has requested David to be his nursing assistant because he is especially good with this patient. At the beginning of today's shift, David approaches Eliza when she is doing the scheduling and mentions that he has provided care for this aggressive patient the previous two weekends and would like a different assignment. When Ralph arrives shortly after, he is dismayed to see that Eliza has already assigned David to work on another unit. He marches over to Eliza and angrily asks, "What do you think you are doing? I need David with me!" Eliza tells him that she promised David that he could work on a different unit. Ralph throws up his hands and walks away while he says, "This is a ridiculous way to make staffing decisions!"

Discussion Questions

1. How would you describe Eliza's leadership style? What problems might this contribute to, and what would you suggest she do differently? Are there any implications regarding how she delegates?

2. Describe the conflict between Eliza and Ralph. Create a dialogue between them that would demonstrate respectful listening and assertiveness.

3. Are there any concerns about this situation that might warrant conversations involving Ralph, Eliza, and other leaders in the organization? What suggestions do you have?

SUMMARY

Communication and emotional intelligence are woven into the fabric of leadership development. By choosing a career in nursing, students are already on a leadership path. Wherever students take their nursing careers, their ability to act as effective leaders, including delegating tasks and managing conflicts, will help ensure safe and quality care, healthy workplaces, and satisfying work.

Reflection Questions

1. What leadership style seems most comfortable to you? Think of an example when you have used this style in a leadership role as a student nurse.

2. Which is harder for you: leading or following? What is it that feels more uncomfortable about the other?

3. Think of a conflict you have had with a fellow nursing student. How might this affect your role in working together on a team? What could you do to address the conflict? What kind of support might be helpful?

References

American Nurses Association Leadership Institute. (2013). Competency model. Silver Spring, MD: American Nurses Association. Retrieved from www.ana-leadershipinstitute.org/Doc-Vault/About-Us/ANA-Leadership-Institute-Competency-Model-pdf.pdf

American Nurses Credentialing Center. (2014.) Magnet Recognition Program model. Retrieved from www.nursecredentialing.org/Magnet/ProgramOverview/New-Magnet-Model

Burns, J. M. (1978). Leadership. New York: Harper & Row.

Crowell, D. M. (2011). Complexity leadership: Nursing's role in health care delivery. Philadelphia: F. A. Davis Company.

Education Career Articles. (2013). Nurses: Advice for conflict management. Retrieved from educationcareerarticles.com/career-information/career-news/nurses-advice-conflict-management

Goleman, D., Boyatzis, R. E., & McKee, A. (2013). Primal leadership: Realizing the power of emotional intelligence. Boston: Harvard Business School Press.

Greenleaf, R. K., & Spears, L. C. (1977). Servant leadership: A journey into the nature of legitimate power and greatness. Mahway, NJ: Paulist Press.

Hassmiller, S. B., & Truelove, J. (2014). Are you the best leader you can be? Leadership resources for every nurse. American Journal of Nursing, 114(1), 61–67.

Institute for Healthcare Improvement. (2014.) The IHI Triple Aim. Retrieved from www.ihi.org/Engage/Initiatives/TripleAim/Pages/default.aspx

Institute of Medicine. (2011). The future of nursing: Leading change, advancing health. Washington DC: National Academies Press.

Kilmann, R. H. (2011). Celebrating 40 years with the TKI assessment: A summary of my favorite insights. CCP Author Insights. Retrieved from www.cpp.com/PDFs/Author_Insights_April_2011.pdf

Kilmann, R. H., & Thomas, T. W. (1977). Developing a forced-choice measure of conflict-handling behavior: The MODE Instrument. *Educational and Psychological Measurement, 37*(2): 309–325. Retrieved from www. kilmanndiagnostics.com/developing-forced-choice-measure-conflict-handling-behavior-mode-instrument

Sherman, R., & Pross, E. (2010). Growing future nurse leaders to build and sustain healthy work environments at the unit level. *Online Journal of Issues in Nursing, 15*(1), Manuscript 1.

Thomas, T. W., & Kilmann, R. H. (1974). *The Thomas-Kilmann Mode Assessment.* Tuxedo Park, NY: Xicom, Inc.

Epilogue: From Theory to Practice

Thank you for considering the research, strategies, and insights presented in *Successful Nurse Communication*. In writing this text, part of my mission was to create a foundation for understanding the cause-and-effect links that tie effective communication and professional behaviors—including assertiveness, respectful listening, self-awareness, and respect for self and others—to the solutions to problems related to patient safety, workplace violence, and excessive stress. Sometimes these links may be difficult to see, quantify, or change in the midst of relentless and urgent demands on your time. But they are there, and I urge you to look for and attend to them with curiosity and ownership by reflecting on the following questions:

- How might I be contributing to this situation?
- What might others with different perspectives have to share?
- What could I do differently, or what ideas do I have for improvement?
- What might I ask others to do or not do?

By asking yourselves these questions and carefully considering the answers, you will likely be making important contributions to the healthy functioning of your workplace culture and all care-related outcomes.

I envision you, individually and collectively, participating in healthy dialogue with colleagues, leaders, and patients—dialogue that will transform healthcare systems into dynamic learning organizations where empowerment, respect, ongoing learning, and the safest, most compassionate care are ingrained in the culture.

I hope this text will help you to increase your ability to practice safe, effective, patient-centered, timely, efficient, and equitable care; to thrive professionally; to treat yourselves and others respectfully; and to ask for the support you need and deserve.

The job of applying the material in this book to your continuing education and eventual practice is ongoing. I hope this text remains a resource and has given you skills for *Successful Nurse Communication* as well as the wisdom to appreciate its importance.

INDEX

Page numbers followed by "f" denote figures